# WEIGHT CONTROL IN PREGNANCY

Based on the most up-to-date research, this book shows how it is possible to control weight, and the cravings associated with pregnancy, safely and successfully – resulting in excellent health for the mother and the birth of a healthy baby.

GW00724730

# WEIGHT CONTROL IN PREGNANCY

## Healthy Mother – Healthy Baby

*by*

## Dr Jennifer J. Ashcroft and Dr R. Glynn Owens

THORSONS PUBLISHING GROUP
Wellingborough * New York

First published 1986

© JENNIFER J. ASHCROFT and R. GLYNN OWENS 1986

*All rights reserved. No part of this book may be reproduced or utilized in any form or by any means, electronic or mechanical, including photocopying, recording or by any information storage or retrieval system, without permission in writing from the Publisher.*

British Library Cataloguing in Publication Data
Ashcroft, Jennifer J.
 Weight control in pregnancy: healthy mother—
 healthy baby.
 1. Pregnant women—health and hygiene
 2. Reducing
 I. Title II. Owens, R. Glynn
 613.7'045      RG525
 ISBN 0-7225-1189-2

Printed and bound in Great Britain

## Dedication

To Barrie, Chloë, Henry and Lizzie

# Contents

# PART 1

# What You Need to Know
# Before Starting

# 1

# Pregnancy:
# A Time for Full Physical Health

**Healthy pregnancy leads to healthy baby AND slim, fit mother**

This book is written for the woman who wants to do all she can to ensure for herself a safe and healthy pregnancy, a pregnancy which results in two things:

1. the birth of a healthy baby
2. the best possible health for the mother, both during the pregnancy and after the birth.

We are going to describe, in detail, just how to achieve both of these aims. It will involve eating the right kinds of foods (and not putting on more than the amount of weight recommended by your doctor). And it will also involve developing healthy habit patterns, such as when best to exercise; when best to relax.

You are NOT going to be told to follow some strange or cranky diet. Nor are you going to be told to go against your doctor's advice in any way. Rather, we are going to tell you about the most up-to-date research on nutrition, exercise, relaxation, and other factors related to a healthy pregnancy. AND we are then going to tell you just how to put all this good advice into practice.

You will be shown what extra nutritional demands pregnancy places on you, and also what kinds of food to eat to obtain these essential nutrients. Your doctor will advise you to eat well. We will show you just how to do this. Many ante-natal clinics tell you not to add more than 20 lb (9 kg) to your weight when pregnant. Other clinics might suggest a *little* more. But no one would advise a weight gain of more than 28 lb (13 kg). Whatever your clinic's advice, this book tells you what it means – how much weight is likely to be baby, or associated directly with the pregnancy; and, unless you are careful to avoid it, just how much weight is likely to be unsightly fat deposited on you, and that will be there after the birth! In case you're worried about how to eat right when you are suffering from morning sickness, we explain exactly what causes this, and how to eat to minimize that sick feeling so many women suffer from in the early months of pregnancy. If you're worried about cravings for certain foods, we discuss these too, and how to handle them.

There will be times when you feel tired – we show you how to relax. But it is important to know that doctors nowadays recommend, for most women (unless suffering from certain medical conditions, for example, high blood pressure; threatened miscarriage), that exercise *is* beneficial. We tell you how to exercise in the best possible ways for pregnancy. And you won't find it too difficult either. A recommended 30-minute walk can be far less of a strain on the legs, and far more enjoyable, than 30 minutes standing at the kitchen sink doing the washing-up. Not only can walking be more pleasurable, it's also far healthier. This is because standing on one spot helps promote the development of varicose veins, whereas walking will have the opposite effect. The leg movement involved with walking actively helps prevent varicose veins developing in the legs!

So, what does having a baby mean for *you*? Many women feel that although they really want a baby, they must pay a price. And that price is their own permanent physical change, for the worse. Once pregnant, many women think that their slim, youthful shape is gone, not only whilst carrying the baby, but forever afterwards too. They might think it is impossible, or abnormal (or at least very unlikely!) that they will regain their figure. THIS IS TOTALLY WRONG. A 'motherly' figure need not be the same thing as a fat figure. *If* you follow current medical advice, as outlined in this book, *pregnancy will mean*:

1. producing a healthy baby;
2. *not* finding the pregnancy a misery because you are burdened with lots of excess fat, or because you are constipated, or get varicose veins. You should enjoy the pregnancy;

3. *not* having stretch marks over stomach and thighs (often caused by gaining more than the recommended amount of weight);
4. regaining the slim figure you had before you were pregnant;
5. looking as good in a bikini (or whatever type of beachwear you prefer!) after the birth as you did before;
6. having a lot more energy to play with your new baby!

## Before the pregnancy: a few things that will help if you get the chance to do them

If you are already pregnant, you may not wish to read this part and may go straight on with Chapter 2. However, if you smoke, read the section on smoking (page 17). And if you enjoy alcohol, read the section on alcohol (page 20).

It is true that having a baby places an extra load on the mother – in more ways than one! Not only does she weigh more, she needs to eat more, and goes through a whole range of physical and emotional changes. But before we describe all these changes in detail, it is worth spending a few moments considering the physical condition the woman is in *before* the pregnancy even begins.

The timing of some pregnancies occurs with meticulous planning. Thanks to modern contraceptive methods we can usually choose when *not* to have children. (Of course, actually managing to conceive a child at a certain date is a much chancier business. It may take several months or longer, trying to get pregnant, before you actually succeed!) However, let us assume you are planning to stop using contraception in the near future, let us say six months or so from now. Is there anything you can do to promote maximum physical fitness in readiness for becoming pregnant?

Yes, there are several things you can do. Although, if you are suffering from some serious problem (for example, you may be very overweight; or you might think you are heavily dependent on certain drugs, such as alcohol), or if you are suffering from some kind of illness, you must consult your doctor. Tell him or her about your particular difficulty, and mention, too, that you feel it is important to discuss your problem with a view to doing something about it *before* you try to have a baby.

Most women, though, are in a reasonable state of health.

However, this does not mean that there is nothing that can be done in order to prepare for pregnancy. The first thing to do is to take stock of some major factors, all of which are extremely important:

1. diet and weight. Is your diet a healthy one? How much do you weigh? Are you overweight, underweight, or just about right?
2. how much do you exercise? What kinds of exercise do you do?
3. do you smoke? How many a day?
4. do you drink alcohol? How much?

Let us take each of these four factors in turn:

### 1. *Diet and weight before pregnancy*

What kind of food do you eat? Most women eat a standard type of diet; two, or perhaps three square meals a day, with the odd snack (a biscuit or some chocolate, a piece of cheese, or a slice of toast) as well. The average Western way of eating is now recognized to be not quite as healthy as was once thought. Medical opinion is that we tend to eat too much fat, too much sugar, and too much salt. Generally, we would *all* be much better off if we cut down on these three items. And we would benefit if we compensated by eating more fibre-rich food, such as fruits and vegetables (especially peas and beans) and wholegrain cereal products. This is just a brief outline of a healthier way to eat for everybody, not just pregnant women! A much fuller description of what to eat for maximum health is given in Chapter 4.

Next, how happy are you with your weight? If you are really obese, you need medical help. Most women do not fall into this category, however. They may think they are a little overweight, maybe 10-20 lb (4½-9 kg), or perhaps a little more. Most women will occasionally go on some kind of diet or other. They may restrict fats, or count calories, eat special kinds of foods, or try any one of the many and varied weight-reducing methods so widely advertised in magazines and books. It's not so unusual to go on a diet and lose some, or even all, of your excess weight. But keeping it off is a different matter. Some women are very successful with this and we offer them hearty congratulations. But statistics suggest that about 9 out of every 10 dieters find that the weight creeps on again as they resume their old eating habits. It does not matter which diet is followed, weight loss by going on a diet is nearly always regained when the diet is finished.

So, what lessons can be learnt from this? Ask yourself, do you fall into the category of the 'yo-yo' dieter? That is, do you lose a little weight, then put it back on; lose a little again, only to regain it shortly after? If this is true for you, then what we suggest is that you stop 'going on diets' once and for all. Instead, we would like you to lose weight by changing your everyday eating habits permanently. This does *not* mean that you give up cake or sweets or biscuits or *anything* that you really enjoy. Rather, we are going to show you how to take a fresh look at restructuring your whole approach to eating, to make your life, and your baby's life, a healthier one. We will tell you what kinds of food are best and what to eat in moderation. We will also teach you strategies you can use to make the healthy changes to your eating patterns permanent. The basic behavioural strategies described in Part 2 of the book can be used whenever you wish; use them to help you guide and monitor changes you will want to make to your eating and exercise habits.

Most women won't be losing fat at all during their pregnancy. It is very difficult to ensure adequate nutrition for you and your baby if you are trying to severely restrict your food intake whilst pregnant, so it makes sense to lose unwanted fat BEFORE pregnancy. We will be explaining later how to control what you eat so that you keep to the medically recommended amount of weight gain in pregnancy. But this entails eating nutritious foods and not gorging yourself on poor quality foods. We are *not* talking about dieting in the way most women use the word, to mean severely restricting overall calorie intake by some method of food deprivation.

There is no reason, however, why you should not lose weight slowly, perhaps 2 lb (1 kg) a month, before and also after your pregnancy, if necessary. Simply changing your eating habits (eating in the way that we recommend), and increasing the amount of exercise you do, will help you shed unnecessary fat. The control strategies we will teach you will show you how to balance your food intake and exercise to control your weight exactly how you please, whether pregnant or not. However, you might think that losing 2 lb (1 kg) in a month is just too slow. But do you realize that many women diet, then regain weight, and continue to repeat this cycle for the *whole* of their adult lives? If it takes a year to lose your surplus fat, this is a comparatively short time compared with the decades you will have left to live with neither dieting nor weight problems.

If you are the correct weight for your height there is still plenty you can do to improve your everyday eating habits, as we will show you in Chapter 4. Similarly, this chapter will be useful for you if you are underweight. Healthy eating behaviour coupled with appropriate exercise is the thing to aim for. Some women who are very underweight or undernourished will find it difficult to conceive a baby in the first place. It is then especially important for such women to attain better health so that they can conceive and then support a baby developing within them.

## 2. *Exercise before pregnancy*

Sport is something that, until recently, most people stopped doing as soon as they left school. We are now recognizing the importance of exercise in society generally. Pregnant women are no longer treated like invalids and are advised (unless suffering from some medical complication) to enjoy exercise during the nine months they carry their baby. Obviously, some types of exercise are more suitable than others, and we will be going into this in some detail later.

But *before you become pregnant* is a very suitable time to review and improve on your daily exercise. First of all, increase the amount of activity in your everyday life, in a way that suits you best. For example, you might climb stairs rather than take a lift. Try to go outside for a walk at least once a day, even if it is only to the local shops. And when you *do* walk, do not amble slowly along but stride out; try to get a little out of breath.

Secondly, now is the time to find a sport which you think might be fun (you are less likely to give it up if you enjoy it!). There are lots of things to choose from. Jogging is becoming increasingly popular. Try to make a pact to go jogging with a friend on a regular basis. Swimming is also an excellent exercise. If you can't swim, local baths usually run courses of lessons for beginners of all ages. Basically, you know yourself what you may be likely to enjoy, and you also know what you won't want to try (even if someone were to pay you to do it!). Go for what is likely to give you most pleasure. Perhaps you are not a sporty type though. You are still likely to walk outside your front door, so plan some interesting walks. There are also dozens of books and records available on keep-fit exercises to do indoors. Give it a go. Try to get fit before you are pregnant. Then, when you are pregnant, the aim will be not necessarily to improve on this level of fitness, but to maintain this level in ways that we will explain to you later in the book.

3. *Smoking: some tips on when and how to give it up*
(You can skip this section if you do not smoke!)
It doesn't matter how much you smoke, five, ten or fifty a day, it's doing you harm and it will certainly cause damage to your baby when you are pregnant. Some women find they don't want to smoke when they actually are pregnant. However, you cannot guarantee that this is going to happen to you, so the best time to tackle this particular problem is now. Smoking is bad for you now, it will affect the baby while you are carrying it, and if you smoke after the birth, it will continue to affect your child when it inhales air contaminated by your cigarette smoke.

If you think you might have some trouble giving up smoking, perhaps you should consider the results of research about the dangers of smoking when pregnant:

(a) your baby will receive nicotine and other harmful products such as carbon monoxide
(b) your baby will develop fewer cells in the brain; this effect is permanent
(c) your baby's growth will be retarded
(d) there is an increased risk of still birth or death in early infancy.

The first three things listed are certain to happen if you smoke whilst pregnant. If you are lucky the fourth won't occur: it is estimated that 1 baby in every 100 born to a mother who smokes dies because of damage caused by the mother smoking whilst pregnant.

There are various strategies for giving up smoking. The most successful method seems to be the sudden stop. Pick a day sometime in the near future when you think you will be ready for the change. Make it a time when you won't be under any significant stress, such as moving house. If you know that you always like to smoke on social occasions, do not pick a social time (like Christmas for example) as the time to stop. Having chosen the day on which you are giving up smoking forever, tell people what you are planning to do. Gather support from those near you.

Next, plan some rewards for stopping. Just what are you going to do with the money you save when you stop buying cigarettes? Why not save it up, and every week or 2 weeks or month, take the little lump sum and spend it on a treat for yourself. Or, alternatively, work out how much you could save if you kept your cigarette money for 6 months or a year. There should be enough for a holiday or a visit to a health farm.

Of course, you know that there are likely to be times when you are sorely tempted to start smoking again. Plan some strategies that you might use to counter these moments. Make out a list of things you think might work for you. Some people find that chewing gum, or peeling then eating some fruit, helps. If you are at home you can go and have a bath, or keep your hands busy with knitting or sewing. It is up to the individual to decide on the ways that are most likely to work in her own particular case.

Maybe you've tried just giving up, and it didn't work. What should you try next? Perhaps you are more likely to take your campaign seriously if you know you will damage your baby if you smoke whilst you are pregnant. Perhaps your previous attempts to stop smoking have failed for a number of reasons. You may have lacked a good enough incentive, like being pregnant. Or perhaps you did not give yourself enough rewards, like treating yourself with the money you would have spent on cigarettes. So, give this method of stopping another go. Don't forget, it might mean life or death for your baby.

However, it might be that to stop smoking suddenly is just not the method for you. There are some alternative ways. You can buy anti-smoking tablets at the chemist. Or perhaps your doctor might suggest nicotine-based chewing gum. But it must be stressed that these are only an *aid* to your own campaign to battle against cigarettes.

You might always try cutting down gradually on the number of cigarettes you smoke. Keep a diary for a few days and record, for each cigarette, the time of day it was smoked; what you were doing whilst you were smoking it (activity); where you were (place); and rate how important that particular cigarette was to you. For the rating use a 1-10 scale, where 1 is not at all important, and 10 is as important as could be.

A typical day's diary might look like this:

### DAY 1: MONDAY

| time | activity | place | rating of importance |
|---|---|---|---|
| 8.00 am | drinking coffee | kitchen | 10 |
| 8.30 | just finished breakfast, having coffee | kitchen | 8 |
| 8.45 | just finished breakfast, having coffee | kitchen | 6 |
| 10.30 | having a chat with a friend | lounge | 7 |
| 10.40 | having a chat with a friend | lounge | 9 |
| 10.50 | having a chat with a friend | lounge | 5 |
| 1.30 pm | just finished lunch, having coffee | kitchen | 8 |
| 1.40 | just finished lunch, having coffee | kitchen | 4 |
| 3.30 | having a coffee | lounge | 8 |
| 3.45 | having a coffee | lounge | 3 |
| 5.00 | reading a magazine | lounge | 5 |
| 6.00 | talking on the phone | hallway | 8 |
| 6.10 | talking on the phone | hallway | 7 |
| 7.30 | just finished dinner, having coffee | lounge | 8 |
| 7.45 | just finished dinner, having coffee | lounge | 4 |
| 9.00 | watching television | lounge | 6 |
| 10.00 | having supper | lounge | 8 |

After a few days or a week, some pattern should emerge. You will find there are certain cigarettes you really need, for example, the first of the day, before breakfast, is extremely important to many people. Others may find that smoking is very important whilst having a drink with friends, or if they are socializing in a pub or at a party. What you should do is try and manage without those cigarettes you find least important (the ones you rate lowest in your diary). Cut down by as many as you comfortably can, even if it is only one less a day. Stay at this level for a while, until you are happy with it, then cut out one cigarette more. Continue with this method until you reach 0 cigarettes a day. Go as slowly as you like;

if it takes you a year to give up, it is a job well done. Don't, if you can help it, become pregnant whilst you are going through this process. Wait until you've given up smoking completely. This will ensure the safety of your baby AND it will be easier for you to focus on your weight control without having to worry about other habits as well.

Many smokers find that they can reduce their cigarette consumption to about ten a day using this slow method. Then each of those ten is really important to them and they find it difficult to drop below this number. But remember that smoking only ten cigarettes a day will cause damage to your baby if you are pregnant. So these ten do have to go. Try sticking to ten a day for 2 or 3 months, until you comfortably feel you are not a heavy smoker. Then, you have two courses open to you. Either you can resume the method you were using all along, cutting down one cigarette at a time (nine a day for a month; eight a day for the next month; and so on), or you could adopt a different strategy. Having become a ten a day smoker, you could then try the 'clean break' method we described first. You go straight from being a ten a day smoker to a non-smoker. You pick your day for stopping, and then you STOP.

If you are a smoker, *and* you are already pregnant, do not despair. To avoid causing harm to the developing baby, give up smoking by the time you are 4 months pregnant. Most of the damage seems to be done between the fourth month and birth, so there is still time to quit if you pick a fast method to stop smoking.

### 4. *Alcohol: is it safe?*

This is a very controversial matter at the moment. Some authorities claim that a *little* alcohol is not likely to be harmful whilst you are pregnant. Others say it is best to do without entirely. However, *all* would agree that heavy drinking is a big mistake and is harmful to the developing baby (and also to the mother, of course!). So, if you have an alcohol problem, do something about it now. Luckily, there are many organizations that your doctor will direct you to if you need help with alcohol addiction. If you consider yourself a moderate drinker (you drink socially, a little on most days), you might consider reducing the amount you consume whilst pregnant. Avoid hard spirits. You might enjoy a single glass of wine with the occasional meal, but don't make a habit of it. Don't drink alcohol everyday. Don't drink alcohol on an empty stomach. But if you want to be absolutely safe, avoid alcohol entirely, from the time of conception of the baby. Avoiding alcohol, especially in the first 13 weeks, probably won't be as difficult as all that, as a great many women find that once they are pregnant, they find the very thought of an alcoholic drink makes them feel sick. So, by avoiding alcohol during pregnancy, you are playing safe with regard to the well-being of the baby. And, importantly, you are avoiding a drink which is of very little value from the nutritional viewpoint. Alcohol is going to be of no benefit in aiding the development of your child, and in keeping you healthy and at the appropriate weight.

# 2

# How Your Body Changes

There are very many changes that occur to you during pregnancy. Some of these are extremely obvious, of course, such as the increasing size of the abdomen. However, there are a great many internal changes to your own functioning that are not so obvious. For example, did you know that the volume of circulating blood increases by as much as 40 per cent? Or that your heart beats faster? Or that your lower ribs change position, flaring very slightly outward to accommodate the baby? We are not going to give you a detailed, medical account of every tiny change brought about by pregnancy. This would be very lengthy and complex, and far beyond the scope of this book. Rather, we are going to describe some of the major changes that occur, and that we think will be of interest to you in understanding some of the effects of pregnancy you may notice in yourself.

We are going to describe how you are likely to feel, and changes you will probably notice, as you progress through the pregnancy. To do this we have divided the total 40-week pregnancy into three major parts, or trimesters as they are called. The first trimester covers the first 13 weeks of pregnancy; the second trimester refers to weeks 14-28; and the third trimester is from week 29-40, when the baby is actually born. Some of the changes or symptoms of pregnancy only usually occur at a particular period during the 40 weeks. For example, a feeling of sickness, in most women, would not be present after the 13th or 14th week. However, some of the symptoms (such as constipation) might occur at any time. And some changes (such as darkening of some parts of the skin) might start fairly early on and then continue throughout the pregnancy. Also, there is a certain amount of variation from woman to woman. Or, indeed, the same woman might find, if she has more than one child, that the symptoms she experiences during her pregnancies are somewhat different. For example, she might not suffer from sickness at all with one pregnancy, but then might with another. Some women find they feel sick through most of their pregnancy, but this is rare. It is generally an early symptom only. So, you can see that you must take the following description of changes during pregnancy only as a guide. It is there to give you some indication of what *generally* happens, and when it happens, to most women when they are pregnant.

## The first trimester (weeks 1-13)

Pregnancy is counted from the first day of your last period before conception. The baby is actually conceived about 2 weeks after this date. Therefore, although the pregnancy is officially 40 weeks, the time from conception to birth is 38 weeks in total. From conception (end of week 2) until the end of the first trimester (week 13) is a very important time, as the tiny embryo (the fertilized egg) develops from being so small that it is invisible to the human eye, into a small but fully formed human being. At the end of the first 13 weeks the baby is about 3 in (7½ cm) long and weighs 1 oz (28 g).

What happens to you during the first trimester? The first thing you will probably notice is that your period fails to arrive at the end of week 4. Occasionally, there may be a slight blood loss when the period is due, but nevertheless, as you are pregnant, this blood loss stops, and the baby continues to develop inside of you. If you do suffer blood loss during pregnancy, it is wise to mention it to your doctor and follow the advice you are given.

One of the first things often noticed is a sensation of sickness. This does not necessarily mean actually being sick. Only rarely do women feel so bad that they take to their bed, unable to continue with day-to-day activities. Extreme nausea will need medical advice. But most women will feel sick just for a small part of the day (when this is early and involves vomiting it is termed 'early morning sickness'). Many women, though, just feel slightly queasy for some of the day. It may be morning, afternoon, evening, or any combination of these three times. They may feel that certain foods or drinks make them feel ill. Common examples are fatty foods, very sweet foods, coffee, strong tea, and alcohol. Women who normally like coffee and cake in the afternoon might suddenly find the idea repulsive. Some may have liked big meals with fatty meats and sauces, washed down with a good wine, but when pregnant, in the first trimester, the very thought leads to a feeling of sickness.

The good news is that you can help matters considerably by avoiding these things that make you feel sick and eat the foods you now enjoy instead. Small, frequent meals help. You may also start to long, or crave, for food you never enjoyed before. So, generally, your eating habits are likely to be turned upside down. During this first trimester women frequently lose weight. This is not important in the average size woman. As long as the food you *do* eat is appropriate, you have nothing to worry about. We will be telling you later on just how to cope with eating during this stage of the pregnancy.

Changes in the breasts are usually very noticeable right from the time of the first missed period (week 4). The breasts feel much more sensitive and tender. They enlarge slowly but noticeably so that even by the 7th or 8th week you may find your bra feels too small. There is an increase in blood supply to the breasts and you might observe the superficial veins as a fine blue tracery under the skin of the breasts. Small bumps (called Montgomery's tubercles) appear on the areola (the pink area around the nipple), and the nipple itself also enlarges and becomes sensitive. You might also notice, by the end of the first trimester, the beginnings of pigmentation, the gradual increase in colour to brown, which occurs to the nipple and areola during the course of the pregnancy.

You will also find that from about week 6 until week 12, you need to pass urine with greater frequency than usual. This is partly because of the increasing blood supply, causing a certain amount of vascular congestion around the neck of the bladder, and also because the womb is enlarging and pressing on the bladder. After the first trimester the enlarging womb rises up out of the pelvis into the abdomen, thus reducing pressure on the bladder. You will find, therefore, at about week 13, your need to pass urine will go back to normal frequency. (Of course, in the final weeks of pregnancy, especially when the head is engaged, pressing down into the pelvis in readiness for the birth, there is once again pressure on the bladder, resulting in the problem of frequent urination returning.) So, at various stages of pregnancy it is quite normal for you to pass urine more often than usual. However, you should not feel pain or discomfort whilst doing so. If this occurs you must consult your doctor.

When will your pregnancy start to show in terms of your abdomen actually becoming bigger? Well, certainly not in the first trimester. When you are *not* pregnant, the womb is much smaller than most people imagine, about the size of a tangerine. It is situated well down in the pelvis and therefore cannot be felt by placing a hand on the abdomen. The walls of the womb are made of muscle. The womb gets bigger during pregnancy by an increase in size of the muscle fibres. Progesterone, a hormone associated with pregnancy, has a relaxing effect on the muscle fibres, allowing them to grow and stretch. By week 6 the womb begins to change shape, starting to go soft and round. It grows to about the size of an apple by this 6th week, and then to the size of an orange by week 9. At week 12 the womb is the size of a grapefruit and only at about this stage is it large enough to detect the top of the womb rising up out of the pelvis. If a hand is placed on the abdomen and is pressed gently downwards, it should be just possible to feel the top of the womb (called the fundus). The doctor will do this when you go for ante-natal check-ups, to find just how large the womb has become. At the end of the first trimester the womb is still very low down, and in fact, it isn't until week 22 that the top of the womb gets as high as the navel! So, if your abdomen looks like a large round ball in the first trimester, it isn't because it is full of baby in the womb. It is much more likely that it is because your intestines are full of food and you are constipated!

We have mentioned that the hormone progesterone relaxes the muscular walls of the womb, thus allowing it to expand throughout pregnancy. The womb is an example of a particular type of muscle, called smooth or involuntary muscle. That is, it is made of muscle that you cannot move voluntarily, as you can, for example, in your arms and legs. Involuntary muscle is found in other places besides the womb, such as in the walls of the intestine (the gut) and in the walls of the veins. Progesterone acts to relax all the involuntary muscles, not just the womb. This is, in many ways, useful to the pregnancy. If the muscle in the walls of the blood vessels are relaxed, then they can become wider and can therefore carry a larger volume of blood. The blood has many functions, such as transporting essential nutrients from the gut, and oxygen from the lungs, to the developing baby. So an increased volume of blood is a very necessary thing. One unfortunate side-effect of relaxed muscles in veins, however, is that in some people it increases the likelihood of varicose veins, most noticeable in the legs. Such women must do all that is possible to avoid them. And much *can* be done to help prevent this problem. Although, unless you are careful, varicose veins can appear at any point in pregnancy, they are not often associated with the first trimester, but tend to come later. Of course, varicose veins need not only occur in the legs. When they occur around the rectum and anal canal, they are most often called piles or haemorrhoids. Although they are more likely in pregnancy, there is a lot you can do to avoid them, as we will show you later. However, varicose veins are unlikely to be a symptom of early pregnancy, so they will be discussed in more detail when we describe the third trimester.

The relaxation of muscle in the gut wall slows down the movement of food through the gut. This may provide a valuable function in so far as it gives the body a longer time to absorb all the available nutrients from the food before it leaves the body. However, if you are eating the wrong kinds of foods (too low in fibre), or are not drinking enough fluids, or are spending long periods lying down or generally inactive, then there is a tendency for the food to stay in the intestine (gut) for too long. That is, you become constipated. This should be avoided because not only is it uncomfortable for you, it could well contribute towards the development of piles later on. Do not, if it can be avoided, take laxatives. A correct diet high in fibre-rich foods, and appropriate exercise, can remedy the problem in nearly all cases.

From all this you can see that the first trimester is a very important time and a very busy one. The baby may not be large enough to show; your figure will look much the same (although your bust will be bigger), yet there are many changes taking place. These changes are enough to produce a fully formed baby (though small) by the end of the 13 weeks. Obviously, all this is bound to have some kind of psychological effect. You might be more emotional. You might become depressed occasionally, especially if suffering from sickness. At other times you will probably feel elated by the pregnancy. You will almost certainly feel extremely tired during these early weeks. It might be very difficult for others to appreciate just how you feel. You won't look pregnant, you shouldn't have gained weight so won't be suffering from tiredness due to carrying added weight. So, many people might find it difficult to make allowances for you, especially if they have never experienced for themselves the sickness and tiredness so often associated with all the changes of early pregnancy. It is essential therefore that you make it clear to those near to you just how you feel (but don't make a long drawn out case of it and get on everybody's nerves!). Tell them what they can do to help (but don't nag!). And take care of yourself. Don't treat yourself like an invalid. Still continue daily activities, go for walks, do appropriate exercises. But if you feel tired, stop. Sit with your feet up and relax for a while. Go to bed early. Do what you feel your body is telling you to do. And if you have any problems or worries at all, consult your doctor or the ante-natal clinic that is looking after you.

## The second trimester (weeks 14-28)

During this period of the pregnancy the baby continues to grow, and the organs already formed inside its body are maturing. By week 28, the baby is considered viable, that is, if it is born at this stage it would have a chance of survival. It must be appreciated, however, that this chance is a very small one, and depends not so much on the size and weight of the baby but on the maturity of its internal organs. The organs have to be developed enough to take on their full function in helping the baby to survive when outside of the mother's womb.

By week 28 the baby has grown hair on its head and a fine, downy hair all over the body. The whole of its skin is covered with a greasy substance called vernix. This helps protect the skin whilst constantly in fluid: the baby, of course, develops within a 'bag of waters' or amniotic fluid as it is properly called, which is all contained inside of the womb. The baby is 3 in (7½ cm) long and weighs 1 oz (28 g) at the end of week 13. By week 28 the baby has grown to about 14 in (35 cm) and weighs around 2 lb (1 kg).

The second trimester is generally a happy one for the mother. The sickness of early pregnancy has gone. The need to pass urine has returned to a normal frequency; and she doesn't feel as tired. When people say that women 'bloom' in pregnancy, these are the weeks that they are usually referring to. This is also the time that the pregnancy will definitely begin to show abdominally. The womb gets bigger at a regular rate, and by week 16 the top of the womb has reached half way between the pubic hair and the navel. At week 20 the top of the womb is just below the navel, and at week 22 it is at the navel. It then continues to get bigger, and expands upwards at the rate of about the width (not length!) of one of your fingers each week. Not only will you be able to see that you have a definitely rounded abdomen, you will also be able to feel the baby inside of you. This is called 'quickening'. You should begin to feel slight movements at about weeks 18-20 with your first pregnancy, but a couple of weeks earlier with subsequent pregnancies. At first it might be difficult to recognize such movements for what they really are, as to begin with, they are felt only as a fluttering sensation. They do become more vigorous as the weeks go on. You should eventually be able to see your abdomen momentarily change shape as the baby kicks or turns. You might, by the end of the second trimester, also be able to feel your baby hiccuping (although, of course, what the baby is hiccuping is the fluid it is in, the amniotic fluid, rather than air). Hiccupping is felt as a gentle rhythmic jarring of the abdomen every two seconds or so.

The breasts continue to change during the second trimester. Any painful sensitivity you noticed earlier should have decreased, although the breasts will probably still be more tender than usual. At around week 16 a clear fluid called colostrum is secreted and may be expressed by gentle manipulation of the breasts. There is no special need, though, to express the colostrum. By the end of pregnancy you will notice it leaking in small quantities into your bra. Colostrum is the liquid that is present before the milk comes in, after the birth. The areola, the ring of darker skin around the nipple, continues to deepen in colour. You may also notice by week 20 that it appears to get bigger. This is the secondary areola which forms around the areola and helps strengthen the skin in preparation for sucking.

As well as the increasing pigmentation which occurs on the breasts, other areas of skin become noticeably darker. Moles and freckles tend to darken and get bigger. Sometimes fair hair on arms and legs becomes darker and therefore more obvious. The linea nigra is the name for a dark line which starts to appear down the centre of the abdomen at about week 14. It runs from the pubic hair upwards towards (and often a little beyond) the navel. The navel itself also becomes darker. The colour deepens as the pregnancy progresses. Late in the second trimester (and continuing into the third trimester) you might notice the 'butterfly mask' of pregnancy developing. This is an area of light brown colour which spreads from the nose over the cheeks like the wings of a butterfly. The forehead may appear light brown too. This is not at all disfiguring, but makes you look as if you have a healthy tan!

This pigmentation, darkening of certain areas of the skin during pregnancy, tends to be most obvious in dark haired women, and may be far less apparent in fair headed women. In either case, pigmentation tends to fade quickly from nearly all areas (although the areola tends to stay darker) once the baby is born.

During this period the hormone progesterone, as well as causing relaxation of the involuntary muscles, also makes the ligaments and tendons soften. These are special types of cord, with ligaments joining bone to bone, and tendons joining muscle to bone. This softening is obviously very necessary in the pelvic area, where a certain amount of softening and stretching is important in order to make room for the baby, especially at the very end of the second trimester and in the final 3 months of pregnancy. However, ligaments and tendons elsewhere also soften. So, for example, there is a softening of ligaments supporting the spinal column. This might make you predisposed to backache in middle or late pregnancy. But you must note that wearing high-heeled shoes, standing in the wrong way (tending to lean backwards instead of being up straight) and taking the *wrong* sort of exercise, all go towards making the backache worse, or even sometimes causing it. It can be prevented, in nearly all cases, if you take certain preventative measures. Wear shoes with a low heel; comfortable walking shoes, or shoes made for jogging, are ideal.

You can also do exercises to strengthen the back (but don't exercise excessively). Be careful to maintain a correct posture, both when sitting and standing. Keep upright and do not slouch. Make sure your bed is comfortable, with a supportive mattress, definitely not a soft one. And the most important thing is to avoid excessive weight gain as this is sure to be a major contributing factor towards very painful backache.

As your pregnancy progresses you may notice that your gums look slightly swollen and redder than usual. As we mentioned earlier, it is essential for the mother to produce more blood in order to transport all the necessary requirements for growth and development from various parts of her own body to the baby. But this increased blood supply affects many parts of the mother's body. One side effect is producing congestion in the gum area. You might find that your gums tend to bleed a little if you are too vigorous with your toothbrush. Food particles may collect between the swollen gum and the teeth. These can be difficult to remove. Bacteria thrive in these conditions and may infect the gum, making it sore and even more likely to bleed. The teeth themselves may also suffer because of this. Tooth rot during pregnancy has nothing to do, then, with the baby taking calcium from the teeth, as this simply doesn't happen. (It is still important, though, to take plenty of calcium-rich foods, because if there is insufficient in the diet, calcium is taken from the mother's bones to supply the baby's needs.) Bad teeth and problem gums can be avoided by proper cleaning of the teeth and gums with a good quality toothbrush, which is neither too hard nor too soft, and is *not* an old one. Buy a new toothbrush every six weeks. Use dental floss. Don't avoid cleaning the teeth and the gums, even if they are a bit sore. Do consult a dentist, whether you have problems or not. Lastly, a well-balanced diet should not include lots of sugary foods. Avoid them altogether, if you can, to help keep teeth and gums healthy.

During the second trimester, provided you do the right things to ensure the health of you and your baby, you should feel very well. You should be able to keep active. You will have regained your appetite. Food fads may become a little less strong now, and tastes for food may change again. Whereas, in the first trimester, a small meal made you feel quite full, and you didn't want large, fatty, sugary, calorie laden meals, now you may have quite different tastes. Your appetite will probably return and you might want to eat large quantities of food. This is all well and good if the food is nutritious and you do not put on more than 1 lb or so (0.45 kg) a week during the second trimester. Don't 'eat for two'; only a very little extra food is actually required, and if you eat twice as much as you normally eat you will become enormously fat and the baby won't benefit at all. If you get very large because you've gained more than the medically recommended amount of weight, you will increase the probability of suffering for it in the third trimester, with backache, bad teeth, sore gums, constipation, piles, and varicose veins in the legs. You also are likely to get raised blood pressure and suffer severe medical complications which could well affect the health of your baby. We will be describing later just what to eat, and how to eat the right amount to control your weight, during this vital period.

## The third trimester (weeks 29-40)
In this final 3 months the baby continues to grow and mature. In the final 10 weeks fat is laid down under the baby's skin, which gives the baby a rounded look. By the time the baby is born the head hair will have grown to about 1-1½ in (2½-4 cm) in length. There may be a little hair (called lanugo) still left on the body, usually on the shoulders, tops of arms, and perhaps on the forehead. This fine hair had started to grow over the body during the second trimester, but it mostly disappears by the birth. The grease over the skin (vernix) might have rubbed off, or be present in patches, when the baby is born. Babies are nearly always born with blue eyes, but then the colour may start to change shortly after the birth, as the eyes are exposed to light. The average length of a newly born baby is about 20 in (50 cm). The average weight is around 7 lb 8 oz (3.4 kg), although anything from 6 lb 3 oz (2.8 kg) to 8 lb 3 oz (3.7 kg) is regarded as not unusual. On average, boys tend to be 4-5 oz (about 120 g) heavier than girls. Birthweight also has a tendency to increase with each successive child. So usually, a third child is born heavier than the second, and the second is heavier than the first.

During this final trimester, the womb continues to enlarge, the top continuing to expand upwards at the rate of one finger width a week. At about week 36 with the first pregnancy, the womb *drops* four finger widths to where it was at week 32. This is called 'lightening'. It is caused when the baby (which is usually lying upside down) descends, with its head going right down into the cavity of the pelvis ready for the birth (it is 'engaged'). The womb then continues to enlarge, travelling upwards again at the rate of one finger width a week, so that by week 40 it will be back in the same place it was before it dropped. If the pregnancy is not the woman's first, the womb will reach a certain height at about week 36 and then stay there until the head of the baby engages, usually not until labour begins at week 40. The womb (which is, after all, basically a muscular bag) contracts at intervals throughout life. Contractions of the womb become very marked in the third trimester, and are called Braxton Hicks contractions. They occur about every 20 minutes. If you place your hand on your abdomen you will feel a definite hardening that comes when the walls of the womb contract. The abdomen itself will change shape slightly. Occasionally, women do mistake Braxton Hicks contractions for those which occur at the beginning of labour, because of the basic similarity between the two. (However, with labour, the contractions becomes much more forceful and more frequent than every 20 minutes.)

If you have not been careful, you might notice that stretch marks have appeared on the lower parts of your abdomen, and sometimes elsewhere, such as the top of the thighs, and even the top of the arms. These have nothing to do with the kind of skin you have. They occur to a small extent because of the production of pregnancy hormone (progesterone), but mostly they come because of excessive weight gain. If you do not put on more than the minimum recommended weight (around 20 lb or 9 kg) you almost certainly will NOT get stretch marks anywhere. Similarly, provided you keep control of your weight and do the right exercises, the abdominal muscles themselves should not overstretch, and will go back into shape after the birth. Exercises will help. Don't be afraid, even when really pregnant, to pull your abdominal muscles right in. You won't be squeezing the baby as it is well protected inside its bag of fluid. Wearing a girdle or corset will not help you retain muscle tone, but if anything, will make it worse. The abdominal muscles themselves act as a girdle provided you use them correctly. Posture in the third trimester is very important and you must try to stand upright, with abdomen muscles pulling you inwards (some people refer to this as having their 'stomach pulled in'). If you don't take this advice you are going to suffer from all sorts of unnecessary aches.

Towards the end of pregnancy, when the head is engaged or the baby is low in the pelvis, you will once again need to pass water with greater frequency than usual, as you did in the first trimester. You might also find that you occasionally get a sudden and urgent need to pass urine, caused by the baby bouncing suddenly against the bladder.

Although morning sickness doesn't return, you might well have some digestive troubles due to heartburn. This is a very misleading term as it has nothing to do with your heart, although it might feel that way. What you sense is a hot burning in your chest. Progesterone, the muscle relaxing hormone, relaxes the muscular valve at the upper end of the stomach. This allows the acid contents of the stomach to go back upwards into the more delicate tube which leads up to the mouth (the food pipe, or oesophagus as it is named). When the stomach contents go back into the food pipe in this way, you feel a burning sensation that is called heartburn. You are more likely to get heartburn if you have gained too much weight, or if you have very heavy or spicy meals. Heartburn is often most noticeable at night. Don't eat a large meal late at night before going to bed. Sleep with an extra pillow; if you are propped up it is more difficult for the food to travel upwards out of the stomach.

We mentioned earlier that varicose veins can occur early in pregnancy because of the relaxing of the muscles in the walls of the veins. This problem is more likely, however, to occur later in pregnancy. This is partly because the enlarged womb presses on the veins in the pelvis and this tends to obstruct the blood flowing back up the leg veins to the heart. If you want to minimize the effect this has on predisposing you to the development of varicose veins, you should make sure, all through pregnancy, that you do all you can to avoid them. Do appropriate exercise (as we'll describe later). Avoid standing still (if you have to stand in one place, for example, when waiting for a bus, try rising up on your toes, or tightening your calf and other leg muscles, or moving from one foot to another). When you are sitting down, put your feet up. Avoid putting on more than the medically recommended amount of weight (see next chapter). If you are slack with these things and varicose veins develop, they are likely to become much worse in the third trimester. They are also likely to be more of a problem the more children you have. They are unlikely to occur in the first pregnancy, and if they do, will probably be very minor.

If you have not been careful to avoid constipation and excessive weight gain earlier, you are extra likely to develop piles (haemorrhoids) in the last months of pregnancy. As explained earlier, these are varicose veins which occur around the rectum and anal canal. By the third trimester the enlarged womb presses on the large vein at the back of the abdomen, which takes blood back to the heart. Veins in the lining of the bowel lead into this large vein. Therefore, if the womb is pressing on it, this tends to obstruct the flow of blood from the veins in the bowel. These veins therefore become all swollen and twisted, and piles are formed. The presence, in the bowel, of hard, compacted faeces, and straining to pass these, helps to enlarge the varicose veins even more, hence making the whole situation worse.

The body tends to retain extra fluid during pregnancy, and a certain amount is quite normal. A very small amount of swelling of the fingers and a slight softening of the contours of the face because of water retention, is not unusual. Ankles and feet might also appear a little swollen, especially at the end of the day. However, severe swelling is not normal. Excessive salt intake may be partly to blame. Hot weather will also make it worse, as will excessive weight gain. You must consult your doctor if you suddenly have problems with severe swelling, especially if it occurs after week 28. This is because it may be associated with pre-eclampsia, a condition which may occur during pregnancy and which, if it is left untreated, can prove dangerous to mother and baby. Ante-natal care is very much geared to making sure the mother is not developing pre-eclampsia. Ankles are usually checked for swelling. Blood pressure is measured to check that it is not too high. A urine sample is also taken and tested. This is tested for several things but one test is to see if protein is present in the urine. When blood pressure is too high protein becomes detectable in the urine. Pre-eclampsia can nearly always be avoided if the signs are detected early and appropriate measures taken. Follow your doctor's advice to the letter. It will probably include complete rest, and if so, it is absolutely essential you do this. Forget exercise. Rest as much as possible. However, it is worth pointing out that it is medical opinion that in very many cases the onset (usually from about week 28) of severe swelling of ankles, face and hands, and of raised blood pressure can be avoided. This can be done if you avoid excessive weight gain, eat the right types of food, and do appropriate exercise, during the first two trimesters.

If you follow the advice in this book, there is no reason why the third trimester should be a difficult one. If you have only gained 20 lb (9 kg) or so, you will not find it hard to move about and you shouldn't become overtired. You should certainly have *no* problems with everyday activities such as getting dressed (leaning over to put on tights or socks, and shoes) or getting in and out of the bath. The average woman should be able to gain a load of 20 lb (9 kg) and still be able to cope. After all, she knows that in a short time that extra weight will go. Her body will resume its original shape *and* she will also have her baby.

# 3

# How Much Weight and When?

**How much weight should you put on, and when?**
There are two things to consider in deciding how much weight you should put on during pregnancy. These are:

1. the weight directly associated with the pregnancy
2. the amount of fat you add to your own body

If you want to be slim within 2 weeks of the birth you should put on no fat at all. This won't harm the baby, or you. You will be back at the weight you were before you were pregnant within about 12 days after the birth. Your abdomen should be more or less flat at this stage. If you exercise to tone up the muscles, then by week 6 after the birth you will be totally back in shape. If you are breast feeding then your breasts will be slightly larger, but this is unlikely to detract from your appearance.

We are going to take each of the two factors above, weight associated directly with the pregnancy, and the amount of fat pregnant women often put on, and talk about each in detail:

1. *The weight directly associated with the pregnancy*
Obviously, this means more than the weight of the baby itself. You are carrying, as *major* sources of extra weight:

(a) the baby
(b) the fluid it is developing in (the 'waters', amniotic fluid)
(c) the placenta (later called the 'afterbirth')

Besides these three things, parts of the mother's own body will be notably heavier; she will have:

(d)  an enlarged womb and bigger breasts
(e)  extra circulating blood
(f)  a little extra fluid generally distributed in body tissues

All the items listed can be said to be a result of being pregnant. Importantly, they are a *necessary result*; you can get pregnant without getting fat, but you cannot avoid weight associated with carrying the baby, the things necessary for its development, all the extra fluids (in tissues and as blood) and the enlargement of the womb and breasts.

So how much do all these things weigh? There are bound to be slight differences from woman to woman. We all know that babies may vary slightly in weight, and we might therefore expect a slight variation in the weight of the other things too. However, the amount of variation is in fact very slight. There will be no more than a few pounds difference, in total weight gain directly associated with the pregnancy, from individual to individual. These, then, are the approximate weights of the items we have listed:

(a)  baby                               7-9 lb (3.2-4.1 kg)
(b)  amniotic fluid ('waters')         2 lb (0.9 kg)
(c)  placenta ('afterbirth')           1½ lb (0.7 kg)
(d)  the womb will enlarge to          2 lb (0.9 kg) originally it was
                                                 only 2 oz (56 gm)!
(e)  the breasts increase by about 1½ lb (0.7 kg)
(f)  extra blood will be about         4 lb (1.8 kg)
(g)  extra fluid in body tissues       2 lb (0.9 kg)

                   TOTAL     20-22 lb (9.1-10 kg)

On the day you give birth, you will lose the weight from carrying the baby, the amniotic fluid and the placenta. This totals about 11 lb (5 kg). On that day and in the next 3 or 4 days you will lose much of the extra fluids you are carrying in the tissues, and also the blood volume will quickly decrease to normal. So you should lose another 6 lb (2.7 kg) or so in the week following the birth. The womb gets smaller very quickly so that within 12-14 days after the birth it is so small it can no longer be felt in the abdomen. If you breast feed, this actively encourages the womb to return to its original size, faster than if you do not feed the baby yourself. Whilst breast feeding the baby, you should actually be able to feel the womb contracting. Excess muscle protein in the walls of the womb are broken down and may then be used to make protein present in the breast milk. However, whether you breast feed or not, the womb will obviously decrease in size and this will mean you'll lose another 2 lb (0.9 kg). Your breasts will not get any smaller if you are breast feeding. In fact, they will become slightly larger when the milk 'comes in', about 3 or 4 days after the birth.

Within 2 weeks of giving birth you should therefore be within about 2 lb (0.9 kg) of the weight you were before you were pregnant. This extra weight is attributable to the larger breasts and the weight of the milk. If you do not breast feed you should be exactly back where you started. Either way, your abdomen will not be flabby and large: it will be flat, and if you exercise appropriately you should regain muscle tone completely by week 6 after the birth. The rest of you, your bottom, thighs, arms, and those places which show fat easiest, should be slim and trim. This will be the case if you only add the amount of weight directly associated with pregnancy (20-22 lb; 9.1-10 kg).

For those who *do* decide to breast feed, you will find you lose the few pounds of excess weight in your breasts when they return to normal size as you wean the baby. We strongly recommend that you *do* breast feed the baby. Breast milk is the perfect food and has lots of advantages over bottled milk, like helping to protect the baby from infection. Breast feeding will not prevent the rest of your body from getting back into shape. In fact, it will help it along by making the womb contract and using the protein from the womb (as we explained above). And, if by any chance you have added a few pounds of surplus fat, the demands placed on your body by the production of milk will almost certainly help to use up this fat.

We hope that we have persuaded you by now that there are many advantages to only gaining the weight directly associated with the pregnancy, around 20 lb (9 kg). But you are now left with a problem. When should this weight go on? This is where you must be very careful indeed. Do *not* increase your weight early on; it will be fat, not weight directly associated with the pregnancy, that you add. If you put on 20 lb (9 kg) in the first 20 weeks, you will find you are much too fat. Weeks 20-30 are also difficult ones as you'll find you feel very hungry at times and there will be a temptation to throw caution to the winds and gorge yourself. This will do the baby no good at all and could, in fact, cause harm if your excess fat leads to high blood pressure and all the serious complications associated with it.

To make things easier for you we have listed the amount of weight you should aim to put on during various stages of the pregnancy:

*YOUR AIM. Weight gain associated with the pregnancy*

WEEKS 1-10    You should aim to put on no weight at all, but eat well (as we show you in the next chapter) and do *not try* to lose weight. You might just lose a little weight due to feeling sick at times and therefore eating less. Do not worry about this. Do not try to make up for it later on. Take this new, lowered weight as the starting point.

WEEKS 11-14    It is acceptable if you gain no weight at all. If you do gain, it should be no more than 3 lb (1.4 kg).

WEEKS 15-30    Add 1 lb (just slightly under ½ kg, actually 0.45 kg) each week. Be careful during this time not to eat more than necessary to satisfy appetite. Do *not* deliberately try to 'eat for two', that is, much more than you normally would. Only a very little extra is needed, as we will show you in the next chapter.

WEEKS 31-36    Add 1 lb (0.45 kg) each week. You'll find it easier to control your food intake at this stage.

WEEKS 37-38    Weight increase stops towards the end of pregnancy. Your weight should stabilize at about the weight you were at the end of week 36. Do not try to add weight now.

WEEKS 39-40    During these final 2 weeks it is very often the case that women lose weight. Hormone levels drop and this indirectly causes a loss of 2-3 lb (0.9-1.4 kg). This is a sign that you are almost at 'term' and the baby will shortly be born.

This scheme represents a total weight gain of between about 20-22 lb (9.1-10 kg) by the end of week 40. If you gain only the amount of weight associated with the pregnancy you will almost certainly fall within this range. Nobody should be outside of this range by more than a pound or two (1 kg).

Incidentally, if you happen to be expecting twins, do not think this means twice as much weight associated with the pregnancy. Aim to put on no more than 28-30 lb (about 13 kg). As with a single baby, the weight should be gained mostly between weeks 15 and 36.

2. *The amount of fat added to your own body during pregnancy*
It is not at all unusual, or unsafe, to add a *little* fat during pregnancy, just a few pounds (1 kg or so). For instance, you might put on a total of 22 lb (10 kg), thinking that this is all associated with the pregnancy directly, but find, after the birth, that this isn't true. It might have been 20 lb (9.1 kg) associated with your particular pregnancy, plus 2 lb (0.9 kg) of fat which you discover is still left 4 or 6 weeks after the baby has been delivered. A small amount of fat, up to 5 lb (2.3 kg) isn't too bad, and shouldn't be difficult to get rid of, especially if you breast feed for a few months after the birth. The fat will almost certainly go during this time provided you use the basic principles of weight control which we'll explain in Part 2 of the book.

What if you gain 28 lb (13 kg)? If you're lucky, you might have a large baby, and therefore have about 22 or 23 lb (10 kg or so) associated with the pregnancy, and only 5 lb (2.3 kg) of surplus body fat. But it's likely that you had less than 23 lb (10 kg) as pregnancy weight. If you had only 20 lb (around 9 kg) as weight directly associated with the pregnancy, then you will have added 8 lb (3.6 kg) of fat. It's even possible, for example, if you have a small baby, to have only 18 lb (8.2 kg) of pregnancy weight; therefore if you gained 28 lb (13 kg) you will have added 10 lb (4.6 kg) of fat. This is going to be more difficult to deal with. Also, this amount of fat will almost certainly show on you, making you look plump. You'll probably feel a bit depressed by it, and annoyed that your clothes either don't fit or are very tight on you. For these reasons we do not recommend a weight gain of as high as 28 lb (13 kg) during pregnancy.

It is true that some authorities used to set a weight gain of 28 lb (13 kg) as ideal. They considered this to be the weight associated with the pregnancy plus 7 or 8 lb (about 3.5 kg) of excess fat. Fat is, indeed, readily stored by the pregnant woman. Fat can be very useful as a store of energy which you can draw on should food become very scarce due to famine or poverty. It ensures that if food is in short supply after the birth, the mother can use her fat reserves, continue to breast feed her baby, and not starve to death. Breast feeding *does* require that the mother eat far more food than usual. A busy mother might not always have time or the inclination to eat the necessary amount. It can be seen, therefore, that in 6 or 9 months of breast feeding, 7-8 lb (3.5 kg) of fat might well be used up. Nowadays, however, we in the western world are not usually faced with either famine or such severe poverty that we cannot afford enough to eat. Many women bottle feed their baby or if they do breast feed, do not do this for a prolonged period (4 months or more). So all this extra body fat is simply not needed. For most women it is best to avoid adding any fat, if possible.

Of course, there is no reason why you should not breast feed your baby for 6 months or more if you wish. Babies thrive on breast milk. If you feed your baby 'on demand' (when it cries for milk), and let it suck for as long as it wishes (until it stops sucking!) there should be no need for the baby to have any food or liquid besides your own milk. There is a growing trend to encourage mothers to breast feed rather than bottle feed and to postpone the introduction of solid foods to 4 months or preferably later, around 5 or 6 months. This is much healthier for the baby. So, if you feed the baby totally with breast milk for the first 4 to 6 months this is best for the baby. And, *if* you have gained a *little* extra fat (up to 5 lb or 2.3 kg) you should find it goes, with very little effort, whilst you breast feed. If you haven't actually gained any extra fat, but want to breast feed, there is no need to be alarmed. Simply eat more. You will certainly have a very hearty appetite whilst you are producing milk, so this is a golden opportunity to really enjoy some good food. Try to maintain your weight at a stable level if you are happy that you do not need to lose weight.

Medical authorities might vary slightly in the amount of weight they advise the pregnant woman to put on. Some say just the weight directly associated with the pregnancy, 20-22 lb (9.1-10 kg).

Some add on a few extra pounds (1 kg) to this figure to account for the tendency of the body to lay down a *little* fat. But nobody will tell you to add more than 28 lb (13 kg). Some women, of course, do put on much more than this. A weight gain of 40 lb (18 kg) isn't so unusual, and an increase of 50 lb (22.5 kg) or 60 lb (27 kg) isn't unheard of. There is no point in fooling yourself that this is because the baby is large, or because you have a lot of 'water' (amniotic fluid), or because you are retaining much fluid in your body tissues generally. Although some women do indeed have big babies, and do have more amniotic fluid than average, and also retain lots of water in their body tissues, this isn't going to amount to that much extra weight. Anyhow, if you are retaining much extra fluid, this is probably associated with the wrong kind of diet and the storage of excess fat as well. A large baby won't add more than a few extra pounds (1 kg or so) extra to your weight than an average sized one. Nobody should put on more than 28 lb (13 kg) at the absolute maximum. Don't forget, 28 lb (13 kg) is the goal to aim for even if you are having twins! If you put on more than this you will find you've 'lost your figure' after the birth. You'll have to really work at getting rid of this excess fat. This doesn't mean starting a super strict diet based on a very limited food intake after the birth. Use the principles of weight control we will outline later to change your eating and exercise habits, to lose weight slowly and steadily and permanently. Breast feeding will help you lose surplus fat so *do* feed the baby yourself. But you will definitely need to change eating habits and exercise habits too in order to achieve a satisfactory result.

## Examples of how different women might cope with their pregnancies, in terms of weight gain

*Example 1: A woman who is her ideal weight at the start of pregnancy*
This woman might aim to put on 20 lb (about 9 kg) in total. If she is typical of many, she might lose 4 lb (1.8 kg) before week 13 or 14, because of feeling sick and therefore not eating as much as usual. However, she still aims to add only 20 lb (9.1 kg) from week 15 to week 40. She monitors her weight very closely and eats good, nutritious food (and avoids too much sugary or high fat food). She gains 1 lb (0.45 kg) each week from week 15 to week 20. This is

what is recommended. However, from week 21 to week 30, despite trying hard to keep a close watch on the kind of things she eats, she gains slightly more than she ought, and from week 21 to 30 she gains 12 lb (about 5.5 kg). What she must *not* do, if she finds that she has gained a little more over a period than she anticipated, is to try and cut back on food and start losing weight to make up for the added gain. This could be dangerous. It might also be misleading to those looking after her, because if she stops gaining weight in the middle of the pregnancy this might suggest there is something wrong, perhaps the baby is not growing as it should. So, if one week she gains 2 lb instead of 1 lb (1 kg instead of about ½ kg), she does *not* start a drastic diet to lose that extra 1 lb (½ kg). Instead, she resolves *not* to *overeat* and to be extra careful in avoiding cakes, sweets, chocolates, very fatty or very sugary foods. She can still have lots of protein (skimmed or semi-skimmed milk especially), fruits, vegetables, and wholegrain products generally (such as wholemeal bread). She should satisfy her appetite with these types of food. If she doesn't over-indulge in these foods (there is *no* need for her to think she has to eat a great deal of extra food, maybe even if she isn't hungry, in order to satisfy the baby) she should put on only 1 lb the next week. She might therefore, in learning to control her weight well as pregnancy progresses, put on 1 lb (about ½ kg) each week from week 31 to week 36. Her weight then stabilizes, she adds no more, and in fact, there is a drop of 2 lb (1 kg) in week 40, a sign that the baby is due. She is now 18 lb (8.2 kg) heavier than she was at week 1. She has gained no excess fat and returns to her original shape within 2 weeks of giving birth. She breast feeds (so, in fact, her bust is a little larger). She obtains the extra nutrients required for breast feeding by eating more. This doesn't make her put on weight because the food goes towards the production of the milk. When she stops breast feeding the baby she is as she was before she was pregnant. Plus, she has a healthy baby!

*Example 2: A woman who begins her pregnancy a little overweight, say 10-15 lb (4.6-6.9 kg)*
What this woman (or, indeed, any woman) should *not* do is to follow a slimming diet which involves a very limited food intake, whilst pregnant. It will be very difficult, unless she knows an awful

lot about nutrition, or is under strict medical supervision, to make sure she is getting the right nutrients she needs to supply her and the baby. It is true, of course, that she might eat less in the first trimester because of feeling sick (associated with the pregnancy). But in nearly all cases this means a very slight drop in food intake, resulting in just a little weight lost during the first 14 weeks. Usually, no more than about 7 lb (3.2 kg) would be lost in this way. This is very different from most slimming diets which would normally result in about 2 lb (1 kg) lost each week (a total of 28 lb, or 13 kg by the end of 14 weeks). Also, most slimming diets, as well as restricting sugar (which is fine, as sugar has no vitamins, minerals or protein) also restrict other foods. So, for instance, many slimming diets restrict milk to ½ pt a day. This is all right if the woman is not pregnant, but terrible if she is. She is going to need plenty of calcium, and milk is an excellent way of obtaining it, but she'll need more than ½ pt a day. It's therefore best not to eat from a very restricted range of foods. Instead, she should have as much as she likes (enough to satisfy appetite) of high quality nutritious foods, such as very lean meat and fish, low-fat dairy products, soya protein products, bread, rice, spaghetti (all cereal products, preferably wholegrain), fruits and vegetables (especially peas and beans). Fats should be kept to a minimum. Sugar (and foods and drinks with sugar in) should be avoided, as should a high intake of salt and salty foods. A craving for the nutritious foods we have mentioned is something to be satisfied. If the pregnant woman craves for kippers she should have them. If she yearns for a cream bun, she should think again: is there anything else, from the list of foods high in essential nutrients (and low in sugar and fat) that might fill the gap instead? We will be dealing in more detail in the next chapter with just how to eat for maximum health during pregnancy.

The woman in our example is not greatly overweight. Carrying a *little* excess fat at the beginning of her pregnancy is not likely to have a harmful effect, provided she is careful to control her weight in the right way. This woman, because she is a little overweight, should try to put on just the weight associated with the pregnancy, around 20 lb (9.1 kg), with no extra fat at all. Her goal is to put on no weight at all in the first 14 weeks. If she loses her appetite a bit in the first trimester, this should help her to avoid sugary and fatty foods. This might well lead to a loss of 7 lb (3.2 kg) in the first trimester. During the second and third trimesters she uses the techniques of weight control (which will be described later) to add the minimum medically recommended amount of pregnancy weight, 20 lb (9.1 kg). She eats well. Although she is occasionally tempted by a chocolate bar or cake (these, after all, are probably the kinds of food that made her overweight before the pregnancy), she does not binge on these foods. Pregnancy is not an excuse for gluttony. She concentrates on eating more nutritious foods. She knows that if she overeats and adds even more fat to the extra she is already carrying, this could lead to blood pressure problems which might harm her and her baby. So let us say she achieves her goal and adds only 20 lb (9.1 kg) from week 15 to week 40. Now, actually, she lost 7 lb (3.2 kg) in the first trimester, so this means she finishes the pregnancy just 13 lb (5.9 kg) heavier than she started it. She'll lose nearly all of this on the day she gives birth, plus an extra 9 lb (4.1 kg) or so in the first 2 weeks after the birth, She should be about 7 lb (3.2 kg) lighter, 2 weeks after the birth than when the pregnancy started. If she breast feeds the baby, and uses what she knows about weight control in deciding what and how much to eat, and how much to exercise, she should find that it is very easy to lose the little excess fat she is carrying. When she weans the baby she will be her correct weight.

*Example 3: A woman who is slightly underweight at the start of pregnancy*
This woman, if she is the typical skinny type, will probably find it difficult to overeat and become fat, and pregnancy should not pose much of a problem. A realistic goal would be to gain about 22 lb (10 kg). If she adds a little more than this it shouldn't matter so much for this woman, but 28 lb (13 kg) should still be the absolute maximum weight she should gain.

*Example 4: The very overweight, obese woman*
She must seek help from her doctor, who may advise her to add only the weight directly associated with the pregnancy (as with our Example 2 above), or may place her on a special food regime. Close medical supervision is needed for such a woman.

*Example 5: The very underweight woman*

If she is *very* thin, she is likely to be far less fertile and may not conceive a child until she has added a little more body fat. She should eat well on the kinds of nutritious foods we recommend in the next chapter. There is no need for her to overeat on very fatty and sugary products, even if she does want to add weight. However, she does need to increase her daily calorie intake. She should include more complex carbohydrate foods (such as potatoes, bread, rice and spaghetti) in her diet. If she manages to add a little weight and then become pregnant, she should then cope as the woman did in Example 3, described earlier.

If she simply cannot add weight and cannot conceive, she should, of course, consult her doctor.

*Example 6: The woman who puts on much less than 20 lb (9.1 kg) during pregnancy*

This is a rather different kind of example from those we have already given. This woman starts her pregnancy at a certain weight (she might be overweight, underweight, or just right; it doesn't matter in this example). But then she adds only a very small amount of weight during the whole pregnancy, let us say 5 lb (2.3 kg) in total over the 40 weeks. How is this possible, if the weight purely associated with the pregnancy is 20-22 lb (9.1-10 kg)? She must be carrying around this amount of pregnancy weight; the enlarged womb and breasts will be heavier, then there is the extra blood and body fluids, the placenta, the amniotic fluid, and, of course, the baby! This is unavoidable. So in order for the scales to register an increase of only 5 lb (2.3 kg), she must have lost 15 lb (6.9 kg) of her own body fat during the pregnancy. This is too much to lose. Unless she was on a very special diet (probably under medical supervision) she may have been eating far less of certain foods than she needed, and consequently have been running low on some of the essential nutrients. The baby might just be all right; babies tend to take what they need from the mother, provided, of course, it is there to take (that stocks haven't run out entirely). The mother's own body could well suffer though. So, gaining only a *very* small amount of weight in pregnancy is usually to be avoided.

It can be seen from these examples that we never suggest a mother should follow a traditional slimming diet (with severe food restriction) or go hungry during the pregnancy. On the contrary, we are suggesting that she eats better than she has ever done. But we emphasize she eats *better* (foods high in nutritional value, low in sugar). She should *not* overeat, thinking the pregnancy is a good excuse to feed on anything and everything in sight. The pregnant woman will do herself and her baby *no* favours if she puts on more than 20-22 lb (9.1-10 kg). In fact, if she becomes too fat she is much more likely to suffer severe complications which could well harm the baby.

## Advantages of gaining the medically recommended amount of weight and not getting fat during pregnancy

Firstly, what are the advantages, for the baby, of the pregnant mother controlling her weight? The mother, if she follows the advice in this book, will be controlling her weight (putting on 20-22 lb, or 9.1-10 kg) by: eating a wide variety of nutritious foods; avoiding foods high in sugar, excess fatty foods, and excess salt; continuing to exercise throughout pregnancy (unless she has special problems and is advised not to exercise by her doctor).

All of these things are of benefit to the baby. The baby needs to be supplied with many nutrients in order to develop and grow, and the mother following a well-balanced food regime will ensure this. (The way we recommend you eat is based on good medical research and isn't a faddy diet, as you will see in the next chapter.) If the mother avoids sugary foods, doesn't eat large quantities of fat or salt, and if she does some exercise (takes walks; perhaps goes swimming; uses an exercise bike), she is likely not to get fat. She will eat enough to supply all the needs associated with the baby, but not so much that the excess is turned into fat and deposited under her own skin! More than 7 lb (3.2 kg) or so of such fat is likely to contribute to high blood pressure in the mother. This could, unless checked, lead to pre-eclampsia (as we explained at the end of Chapter 2). This is dangerous. The baby might even die. So you can see that controlling weight gain as medically recommended is best to ensure the well-being and safety of the baby.

Secondly, what are the advantages of weight control for the

mother? Obviously, she wants to do the best for her baby, as we explained above. There are many other advantages as well. Pregnancy brings about many changes in the body as we showed you in Chapter 2. Indeed, certain things cannot be avoided (although most of them are not permanent and go when the pregnancy has ended). Unavoidable changes are, for example, the relaxation of the involuntary muscles and softening of ligaments and tendons. Certain areas of the skin will tend to darken. Breasts will feel tender and they will enlarge, as will the abdomen. Tiredness and feeling a little touchy, perhaps being more emotional and sometimes bursting into tears for very little reason, are very common at the beginning of pregnancy, and sometimes in the last trimester too. You will have the inconvenience of having to pass urine more often in the first and third trimesters. Your gums will become slightly swollen and might tend to bleed more easily at times. By the end weeks when you are carrying your maximum pregnancy weight, you might feel burdened and ungainly at times. It could be difficult to get a good night's sleep, especially if your preferred position used to be lying on your stomach! You might have some general digestive problems, feeling a little sick in the first trimester, and later on in the pregnancy perhaps having some difficulty with heartburn.

Some of the things in this list may cause some despondency, but they are not *so* bad. Most women can accept them as a temporary part of the process of supporting and nurturing the developing baby. However, many of the inconveniences long associated with pregnancy can, in very many cases, be avoided by following the advice on food and exercise in this book. Here is a list of the things you can go a long way towards avoiding:

| | |
|---|---|
| 1. digestive troubles such as *severe* sickness, or heartburn | Eating small frequent meals, low in sugar and low in fat will help to alleviate symptoms, although feeling sick can be difficult to overcome at the beginning of pregnancy. With heartburn, avoid lying flat after a meal; prop yourself up with pillows if in bed. |

| | |
|---|---|
| 2. constipation and piles (haemorrhoids) | Plenty of fibre and fluid should help you avoid this kind of problem. Exercise, such as walking or swimming, will help keep your bowel habits regular. |
| 3. varicose veins in the legs | Exercise is important to keep the leg muscles strong and in good tone. Strong exercised muscles will do a better job than support stockings in helping you avoid this problem. It is essential, whenever possible, to avoid standing still; walking is better. If sitting, put your feet up on a stool; do not cross your legs or ankles. Don't gain too much weight. |
| 4. backache | Avoid walking in high heeled shoes. Wear good, supportive footwear. Good posture is essential. A supportive mattress on your bed will be a great help. Do not get fat. |
| 5. disease of the gums and possible loss of teeth | Good dental hygiene and avoidance of sugar will prevent gum disease and loss of teeth. |
| 6. stretch marks | If you don't add more than 20-22 lb (9.1-10 kg) and you weren't more than a little overweight at the beginning of pregnancy, you shouldn't get stretch marks. |
| 7. water retention | You might be carrying a *little* extra fluid in your tissues but you can avoid excess fluid retention (leading to a puffy face, swollen fingers, ankles and feet) by not eating too much salt and avoiding gaining too much weight. |
| 8. signs which lead to pre-eclampsia (high blood pressure, protein in the urine, severe water retention) | Control your weight in the ways we recommend and you're far less likely to develop troubles of this kind. |

| | |
|---|---|
| 9. general body fatness, bigger bottom, fatter legs, arms and face | There is no need to suppose that the whole of your body should blow up like a balloon just because you are pregnant. Apart from your breasts and abdomen you should stay approximately the same. And even your abdomen will stay smaller if you don't add excess fat and you keep good control of your abdominal muscles by exercising appropriately. |

You can see that weight control, by having sensible eating habits and doing appropriate exercise, is just about the best way of ensuring a healthy pregnancy for both you and your baby.

# 4

# Food and Pregnancy

**Extra nutritional requirements associated with pregnancy**
The nutritional requirements discussed in this section are, broadly, those recommended by the Department of Health and Social Security, published in the *Manual of Nutrition,* Ministry of Agriculture, Fisheries and Food, HMSO.

There is no one particular diet associated with pregnancy. Nor is there a special food or nutrient that pregnant women ought to have that non-pregnant women do not have. Basically, you should be choosing from the same types of foods that promote maximum health in any individual, pregnant or not, *but* you should be eating slightly more of certain of these foods than if you were not pregnant. For example, you will need more of some nutrients, such as calcium, of which milk, cheese and yogurt are abundant sources. We will describe the major extra things, like calcium, that you will need in order to support the pregnancy.

*Calories*
You will need extra calories when you are pregnant. But just what is a calorie? It isn't, actually, like a vitamin, or a mineral (like calcium), or a special type of protein or carbohydrate or fat. It is a measure of the energy supplied by food, in fact, *any* food (or drink). Everything we consume, whether it is protein, fat or carbohydrate (or any combination of these three) provides us with fuel for our bodies and gives us energy. It is not surprising, perhaps, that a pregnant woman needs extra fuel to support her and the developing baby. As we have said, we normally quantify the fuel power of any food in terms of calories. You've probably

seen calorie booklets which show you exactly how much energy (that is, how many calories) may be supplied by each kind of food. You know that each day you need a certain amount of fuel just to keep your body ticking over (for example, when asleep) plus extra for general activities, the movement involved in day-to-day living. If you take more than needed, the extra is stored as body fat, which may then be used as a store of energy for any occasion that you don't eat enough to supply you with sufficient fuel. This would be the case if there was a famine. Or, when a woman goes on a slimming campaign, she deliberately is reducing food intake (therefore reducing calories) and so uses her own body fat as fuel.

Ideally, people should eat just the right amount of food to supply calories for their daily energy requirements with none extra that will be turned into fat. If you only ate when you were hungry and did a moderate amount of exercise you shouldn't have weight problems. The difficulty is, of course, people are often tempted by certain foods (appetizing desserts; sugary confections) or drinks (such as coffee with cream and liqueurs) to carry on consuming when the meal could well have ended with a main course, and the real hunger gone. Even so, eating extra shouldn't cause too many problems so long as you wait until you are really hungry again before having another meal. But how many people do this? After a special evening meal not many people will forego breakfast simply because they are not hungry yet.

But let us assume that on most days you are eating just enough to supply your needs. Your weight is fairly stable. If you are an average woman (not pregnant) you will probably need around 2,200 calories a day. If you take very little exercise your daily calorie requirement may be far less than this, perhaps as low as 1,600-1,800 calories to maintain a stable weight. However, if you're very active you might need 2,500 calories a day or slightly more, just to provide you with energy for daily living. When not pregnant, how much fuel do you, personally, need each day to supply your needs? Write down the food you would eat on an average day, and then use a calorie booklet to find the number of calories in each food (and drink as well), and then find the total calories by adding up the scores. This will give you an approximate idea, although your calorie requirements might vary slightly from day to day (because you are more active some days than others).

Generally though, most people keep their weight remarkably stable. You yourself know your own pattern of eating (three square meals a day? or are you a nibbler? or do you have small meals in the day and a large meal at night?). You should also have some idea, if you take an honest look at your food habits, whether you need to eat a great deal each day, or a more moderate amount, in order to keep your weight stable. So you must first assess just how much you normally eat when you are not pregnant. Work out what your daily average calorie intake is, if you like. Otherwise, class yourself, as honestly as you can, as a light, moderate, or heavy eater. If you are only a short person, and you sit at a desk all day, drive in a car to and from work, and take no extra exercise, you will be a light eater. If, on the other hand, you have an active job, you like sports such as swimming or running, and especially if you are a fairly tall person, you will be a heavy eater. If you are somewhere in between these two examples, you will probably be a moderate eater.

How much extra fuel do you need, that is, how many more calories should you have, if you are pregnant? Perhaps the most surprising thing is that you need very few extra calories each day in order to support the pregnancy. In the first trimester you might need hardly any extra fuel at all. This will be especially true if you are normally very active but find, in the first trimester, you spend little time engaged in active pursuits because of tiredness so often associated with the early weeks of pregnancy. Many people will find they need to have no extra calories at all in the first trimester of pregnancy. Although the baby is going through the important formative period, growing from a tiny, fertilized egg into a recognizable human being, this does not require much extra energy. You won't be carrying much extra pregnancy weight as the womb and the baby are still so small. So, whether you classed yourself as a light, moderate or heavy eater to begin with, stay with this level and do not eat more. Instead, the first trimester of pregnancy should be a time when you look at the *quality* of the food you are eating. By avoiding sugary products (such as cakes, biscuits, chocolates, sweets) and substituting more savoury items (such as yogurt, wholegrain cereal and skimmed milk, fruit and nuts, or savoury sandwiches) you will be getting more nutrients from your food, without increasing calories and getting fat. We will be explaining just what nutrients you need shortly in this chapter.

In the second and third trimesters you will still need the extra nutrients but you will also need more food as fuel to supply the extra needs associated with pregnancy. Now is the time when calorie requirements increase. This will vary slightly from woman to woman, but the increase is generally small. Each day, from week 14 to week 40, you should need no more than 200-300 calories extra to the number you usually require when not pregnant. If you originally classed yourself as a very light eater when not pregnant (say 1,600 calories a day to maintain a constant weight), you might need 1,800-1,900 calories a day. You can see that this still isn't a great deal. Pregnancy should not turn a light eater into a very heavy eater because she will get very fat indeed! If, before you were pregnant, you were around average and ate about 2,200 calories worth of food each day, you will need 2,400-2,500 calories now. And if you were a very active person before you were pregnant (needing around 2,500 calories a day) *and* if you stay fairly active during pregnancy, you should need about 2,700-2,800 calories a day.

So most people will need around 200-300 calories a day more in the second and third trimesters. This is certainly not 'eating-for-two'. If you doubled the number of calories to 4,000 or so each day, you would become very fat. This could well endanger both you and the baby. In fact, 200-300 calories isn't very much at all. What quantity of food would supply about 200 calories? A calorie booklet will tell you, but we give you some examples:

200-300 calories could be derived from:
    2 eggs, 1 dry slice bread .............. 280 calories
    or 2 oz (56 g) cheese ................. 240 calories
    or ¾ pt full fat milk ................. 270 calories
    or 1½ pt skimmed milk .............. 270 calories

If you ate food to supply you with the number of calories that were usual for you when not pregnant, plus just one of the above items extra each day, this would be approximately the right amount, in terms of providing fuel, to support you and the baby.

Of course, we are not suggesting that in the second and third trimesters you eat what you did before you were pregnant plus

200-300 calories worth of *any* food. You should continue with the habit you began in the first trimester of making sure your total food intake consists of good quality food, high in nutritious value.

There is no need to worry too much about counting calories. We have talked about them in some detail just to show you how very little extra fuel you actually need when pregnant. We will not be asking you to count calories every single day of your pregnancy! Your weight gain, week by week, will be your best indicator of whether you are eating enough (and not too much!). You might have to readjust your food intake very slightly in order to get the rate of weight gain to that which is medically recommended (given in the previous chapter).

As a final note on calories, if you breast feed your baby you will need about 500 calories extra a day after the birth (that is, 500 calories more than when not pregnant). You can see, therefore, that producing milk takes about twice the number of calories as being pregnant. It is for this reason that breast feeding often uses the few extra pounds of fat which may have been stored in the mother. She may not actually eat as many as 500 calories extra each day. The energy needed for milk production has to come from somewhere, so the mother's fat reserves are used up, making her slim again!

*Protein*
Protein is an essential part of the body; it is necessary for the growth and repair of cells. It is not surprising, therefore, that your need for protein increases when you are pregnant and then if you breast feed.

Where are proteins found? Most people know that meat, fish, eggs and dairy produce (milk, cheese, yogurt) are very good sources of protein. However, protein is also found in important quantities in many plant foods, such as cereal products (like bread, rice, spaghetti, breakfast cereals). Nuts, seeds, and pulses (for example, peas, lentils, beans) are good sources of protein too; this is especially true of soya beans and all their derivatives such as soya meat and soya milk. If you eat a mixture of plant sources of protein, then the quality of the protein can equal that found in animal sources. Mixing a cereal product with a pulse product will give you a good quality protein. Examples are beans on toast; rice and peas; lentil curry and rice; spaghetti and soya meat made into a bolognese. Mixing nuts or seeds with cereals or pulses also increases protein value. For example, in muesli, cereal and nuts are mixed together. You can see from these examples that being a vegetarian need not make it difficult for you to meet the protein needs of pregnancy.

Of course, most people do not usually eat animal food without having a plant food with it. This is a very good idea from the nutritional viewpoint. Protein is made up of basic units called amino acids. You might like to think of these units as different coloured bricks. You need an assortment of bricks of different colours in order to do the job of repairing the old body cells and making new ones. Not every protein food will have all the different colours of brick in exactly the right numbers of each colour that you need. So the best way of ensuring that you get the different colours that you require is to eat a variety of protein foods, preferably in the same meal. In fact, we mostly do this without thinking about it. We often have protein from a cereal product (such as bread) with another protein source. We have already given some examples (such as beans on toast). Other examples would be sandwiches with egg, cheese, meat or fish filling; a risotto; paella; pizza; rice pudding; macaroni cheese; breakfast cereals and milk. Mixing foods in this way is a very efficient method of getting protein. And, in fact, it is likely to be healthier to have slightly less protein from animal sources but slightly more protein from plant sources in each meal than people often do. For example, what if you decide to eat a large omelette (four eggs) for lunch? You will, indeed, consume quite an amount of protein. But you could have just as much protein and, in fact, more of a mix of the 'coloured bricks' (amino acids), if you had a two-egg omelette with peas and a slice of bread. There are also other advantages in consuming plant sources of protein with your meal. They contain considerably more fibre than animal sources. This is especially true of pulses (peas and beans) and wholegrain cereal products. This will definitely help to stop any constipation problems. Adding plant products will give you a wider variety of nutrients (such as vitamins and minerals). And importantly, most plant sources of protein have very little fat. Cutting down on fat is one of the major ways anyone can ensure better health.

It should be relatively easy to be certain that you get enough protein when you are pregnant if you choose from a variety of protein foods at each meal. Mix your proteins as we have suggested. Should you feel like a snack in between meals, rather than have biscuits or a similar sweet treat, choose from more nutritious protein-rich alternatives. Perhaps you could have a small savoury sandwich (but be careful to spread butter or margarine very thinly), or a bowl of muesli and milk, or perhaps an unsweetened yogurt with fresh fruit or nuts chopped into it. However, don't eat these extra snacks in between meals unless you feel genuinely hungry, as they can be relatively high in calories, or 'fuel power' (though no more so than chocolate or cakes!)

*Minerals*

These are inorganic elements such as iron, calcium, phosphorus, magnesium, sodium and potassium. Minerals, although needed in minute amounts, have extremely important functions. For example, calcium is an important part of teeth and bones; iron is necessary for the formation of red blood cells. It is obvious, therefore, that pregnancy brings an increased need for minerals. As we described in Chapter 2, the expectant mother may have about 40 per cent extra blood in her body. Obviously, she will need more iron, not just for the baby but also to help manufacture this extra blood of her own. She will become anaemic if she doesn't have enough iron. Calcium will be needed not only for the mother but also to go towards forming the baby's teeth and bones. Extra minerals will also be needed if the mother breast feeds; for example, the production of breast milk demands a high intake of calcium.

There is no need to worry particularly about all the different types of minerals, and just which foods you have to eat in order to get enough of each one. Minerals are present in many foods, such as the protein foods (plant and animal) that we mentioned earlier, and also in vegetables and fruits to some extent. If your diet is rich in such foods you should have enough minerals.

However, you do need rather a lot of iron, and just to make absolutely sure you have enough, ante-natal clinics tend to give pregnant women iron tablets. Some of these tablets also contain folic acid, a vitamin which is also necessary for the production of red blood cells. (Folic acid is also found in liver, vegetables, cereals and nuts.) You may find these iron tablets cause you no problems at all, but a few women report that they experience either constipation or, in some cases, diarrhoea when they take them. If this happens to you it might be best to continue to take them for a few weeks to see if your body adapts to them and the unpleasant side effects wear off. If they don't, have a word with your doctor. It is possible that a different brand of tablet might suit you better. If even this fails, perhaps you might like to negotiate with your doctor about the possibility of having a diet with plenty of iron-rich foods rather than tablets. We stress, however, that you should seek the approval of your doctor for this.

To make it easier for you to plan an iron-rich diet you should know that pregnant women are recommended to have 15mg of iron a day. Which foods would supply you with this amount? Here is a list which might help you choose the correct types of food. Please note, though, that you will have to choose at least three items from the list each day, as each item contains about 4 mg of iron. The foods in this list aren't the only things that contain iron. There are small amounts in other foods, such as potatoes and eggs. But we have listed the foods very rich in iron that you might eat:

*Foods which give around 4 mg of iron*
1¾ oz (49 gm) fried liver
5 oz (140 gm) corned beef
5 oz (140 gm) any cooked beef
5 oz (140 gm) sardines or pilchards
2¼ oz (63 gm) kidney
1¼ oz (35 gm) shell fish
3 oz (84 gm) heart
1 teaspoon curry powder
10 oz (280 gm) baked beans
2½ oz (70 gm) *dry* beans or peas
2½ oz (70 gm) *dry* lentils
8 oz (224 gm) fresh or frozen peas (boiled weight)
5 oz (140 gm) spinach
4 oz (112 gm) oatmeal (before liquid is added for cooking)
4 large slices of wholemeal bread
1½ oz (42 gm) wheatgerm
3½ oz (98 gm) wholemeal flour

2 oz (56 gm) soya flour
3 oz (84 gm) dry figs
3 oz (84 gm) dry apricots
3 oz (84 gm) sultanas plus 2 oz (56 gm) almonds
3 oz (84 gm) sultanas plus 2 oz (56 gm) brazil nuts
6 oz (168 gm) prunes, weighed dry with the stones in

If you pick three items from this list you will have around 12 mg of iron. You are very likely to be getting 3 mg of iron from other foods that you eat and this will total 15 mg. However, if you want to be extra sure you obtain enough iron, you could always pick four items from the list each day. Try not to pick the same things from the list each day. Pick plant sources of iron as well as animal sources. You can have double portions of some things if you like. For instance, if you like liver you're unlikely to be eating only 1¾ oz (49 gm) at a meal. You're much more likely to be having around 4 oz (112 g), providing you with about 9 mg of iron. You then need fewer things from the list that day to total the required daily amount (15 mg). If you're not very fond of meat you can always pick things like dry figs, or oatmeal (made into porridge, or with dried apricots, nuts and sultanas added and made into muesli), or bread. If you used to really like cake but feel you ought not to have it because of its high fat and sugar content, you could always try picking items from the list (flour, soya flour, sultanas and nuts), perhaps adding an egg or milk, and experiment with your own recipes. There is no need to add sugar if you have plenty of dried fruit in the cake. You might need a little fat, but add the minimum (preferably a margarine high in polyunsaturated fat – read the lid or the tub to find if the margarine is of this type). Then you could always have a slice of this special cake, perhaps with a glass of skimmed or semi-skimmed milk and a piece of fruit, as a complete meal in itself. A useful thing to know, incidentally, is that iron, particularly from plant food, is much better absorbed by the body if it is eaten at the same time as a food rich in vitamin C, such as fresh fruit.

As well as iron, the body has a great need for extra calcium. Just to make sure you are getting enough calcium-rich food, you might like to know the following. When you are pregnant you require about 2½ times the amount of calcium you needed when you were not pregnant. It is recommended that expectant mothers have 1,200 mg a day. The richest source of calcium in most people's diets is likely to be dairy food. Solid cheeses such as cheddar and Edam contain just over 200 mg of calcium per 1 oz (28 gm). (Note that cottage cheese, although very good because it has reduced fat, has much less calcium, around 23 mg per 1 oz (28 gm)). Milk, whether it is ordinary whole milk or skimmed or semi-skimmed, is a very rich source of calcium, giving about 680 mg of calcium per pint. A 5-oz (140-gm) tub of plain yogurt would have 250 mg of calcium. Some types of fish also provide a fair amount of calcium. Sardines have 150 mg per 1 oz (28 gm); canned pilchards have 85 mg per 1 oz (28 gm).

Calcium may also be found, although generally in smaller quantities, in some plant products. Some examples are given below:

*Approximate mg of calcium in each 1-oz (28-gm) portion of:*

| | |
|---|---|
| soya beans | 60 mg |
| broccoli | 30 mg |
| spinach | 20 mg |
| parsnips | 16 mg |
| baked beans | 13 mg |
| dried apricots | 26 mg |
| dried figs | 80 mg |
| almonds | 70 mg |
| brazils | 70 mg |
| enriched white bread | 30 mg (it is standard for white bread to be enriched with calcium; it is in the bread when you buy it) |
| oranges | 12 mg |

These quantities may not seem very great when compared with the amount of calcium in dairy food. But don't forget that with the foods in the list you are likely to be having a portion greater than 1 oz of each item. So, for example, a 6-oz (168-gm) portion of broccoli will yield 180 mg of calcium.

If you are eating a wide variety of protein-rich food, of both plant and animal origin, you should be obtaining enough minerals of all the necessary types. A good insurance is to have at least one pint of milk each day, perhaps two pints if you do not have other types of dairy products and you do not like fish. Perhaps you would like to have a glass of milk as part of each meal? Keep fat levels to an acceptable level by either having skimmed or semi-skimmed milk. If you cannot obtain these, or do not like their taste, pour away the cream from the top of ordinary whole milk. You will then have made it less fatty.

We mentioned earlier that iron is better absorbed from food if vitamin C is available at the same time the iron-rich food is eaten. We therefore recommended that fruit should be eaten with iron-rich foods (although vegetables also tend to be a good source of vitamin C and therefore could be eaten instead of fruit if so desired). As well as vitamin C, fruits and vegetables also contain natural acids and these aid the absorption of calcium. Calcium is also better absorbed if present with protein (this occurs naturally with many foods, such as dairy products, which are an excellent source of both calcium and protein). It can be seen from all this that having a mixture of foods (animal and plant sources of protein, vegetables, fruit) at each meal is very important if maximum absorption of minerals is to occur.

*Vitamins*

Vitamins are present in many foods, in animal and plant sources of protein, vegetables and fruits. Like minerals, we need only tiny amounts of the vitamins, which are necessary for health and growth of cells. Although the need for these substances generally does increase in pregnancy (and when breast feeding), you should be getting plenty if you follow the advice on food that we have already given. Do not decide that you will make extra sure you are having enough vitamins by buying tablets from the chemist or health store. Some of these preparations contain very high doses of vitamins. Although excess may usually be excreted by the body, this is not true of vitamins A and D. Large doses of these can poison you. You really shouldn't need vitamin tablets if you are eating sensibly, but if you really feel you'd like to take them, seek your doctor's advice. This will ensure that they are not of a dangerously high dosage.

The major vitamins are A, the B family, C and D. Vitamin A is found, for example, in apricots, peaches, melon, carrots, tomatoes, spinach and peas. Animal sources of vitamin A are fatty fish such as herring and canned sardines, liver, kidney, dairy produce and eggs. This vitamin is also added to margarine.

There is a whole family of B vitamins, but the major ones, $B_1$, $B_2$ and Niacin are found in plentiful supply in wholemeal cereals, wheatgerm, soya products, peanuts, liver, pork and bacon. Note, though, that pork and bacon are both very fatty and bacon is high in salt, so don't have these too often. Vitamin $B_6$ is found in cereals, eggs, meat (especially liver and kidney) and fish. $B_{12}$ occurs in meat, milk and eggs. It cannot be obtained from any vegetable product, so vegans ('pure' vegetarians who have no animal produce) *must* take $B_{12}$ supplements. In fact, to meet the demands of pregnancy vegans may well need supplements for some of the minerals too, especially calcium, and they should be ultra careful to obtain advice from nutritional experts if they wish to pursue their veganism during pregnancy. Vegans should ask their doctor to put them in contact with a qualified dietician who will be sympathetic to their views. It certainly is possible to maintain a vegan diet during pregnancy. It will also be useful to contact the Vegan Society (their address is in the back of the book) for advice on how other vegan mothers have coped.

Vitamin C is found in plentiful supply in fruits and vegetables, so nobody should have any difficulty in obtaining sufficient of this vitamin.

Vitamin D is especially important in pregnancy, as its presence is needed for absorption of calcium. The body can manufacture its own vitamin D if exposed to sunlight. When skin is exposed to the sun (or ultraviolet light) this vitamin is formed under the skin. However, if you are not outdoors a great deal, or if you are well wrapped up when you are, you will have an even greater need for vitamin D in the diet when you are pregnant. Only fatty fish and eggs are a reasonable, naturally occurring source of this vitamin. It is because vitamin D is not widely available in food that it is also added to margarine, along with vitamin A. However, if you are a vegetarian or vegan, do not feel you can rely on vitamin D in margarine or eggs to supply you with sufficient to meet your needs whilst you are pregnant; 1 oz (28 g) of margarine will only give you about ¼ of your daily requirements. Eating 4 oz (112 g) of margarine, although it might give you enough vitamin D, would give you much too much fat. Margarine is very calorific, and contains no protein, so you shouldn't eat a great deal of it. And, if you are a vegetarian who eats eggs but not fish, you might still find it difficult to get enough vitamin D from this source, as one egg will only give you about one tenth of your daily needs. (A moderate portion of fatty fish, such as herring, kipper, salmon, sardines, would supply enough vitamin D for the day or even more!) So, if you are a vegetarian or vegan, and especially if you are not exposed to the sun a great deal, do seek your doctor's advice about obtaining the necessary supplements to your diet.

## Eating for maximum health

Advice in this section is based on the NACNE report (the UK National Advisory Committee on Nutrition Education), published by the Health Education Council, 1983.

We have now outlined the basic nutrients (proteins, carbohydrates, fats, vitamins and minerals) that a pregnant woman will need. However, if she wishes to obtain these nutrients from foods in the healthiest way, there are some useful hints for her in this section. These recommendations are actually applicable to anyone, so she should find them useful after her pregnancy, and also in planning meals for her baby after it is weaned from a milk-only diet.

*Fats*

People in the western world eat far too much fat. There is no need for a pregnant woman to think she needs extra. In order to keep the amount of fat eaten to an acceptable level, here are some things it is easy to do:

1. Have skimmed milk or semi-skimmed milk. If these are unavailable, pour the cream off the top of ordinary milk and drink what's left. Have cheese and eggs in moderation.

2. Use a low-fat spread, such as 'Outline' or 'Gold'. If you don't like these, or if they are unavailable, have a polyunsaturated margarine, such as 'Flora', used very sparingly. Butter and margarine which aren't marked as polyunsaturated tend to be high in saturated fat. These are therefore to be cut down, as generally, we eat too much saturated fat. Solid blocks of cooking fat, such as lard, are also high in saturated fat, so avoid them. If you must cook with fat, then use a small amount of corn oil, sunflower oil or

safflower oil. But generally, grill rather than fry food. There is no need to add fat to food (such as vegetables) after it is cooked. Use the bare minimum of fat if you find you don't like the taste of food without it.

3. Even very lean meat with no visible fat still has fat in it. However, you can keep fat obtained from meat to a minimum by trimming off all visible fat. You can also avoid very fatty meats and meat products. There is a very high proportion of fat in many of these foods, such as chops, sausages, burgers, pork pies and meat pies generally. Do not use the fat from meat to prepare gravy or sauces. In fact, do not use any type of fat to prepare sauces. Occasionally have poultry (low in fat) instead of red meat.

4. If you are very fond of chips, have them cut very thick as they absorb less fat that way. If buying chips from a chip shop, do not eat the very small, fatty pieces of chips often found at the bottom of the bag.

5. Avoid too many fatty snacks such as peanuts and crisps.

6. Salad creams and dressings (for example, mayonnaise) are very high in fat. Try low fat alternatives, or use vinegar or lemon juice or yogurt to prepare alternative salad dressings.

7. Avoid excessive use of pastry in cooking. Use potato as a topping instead in savoury products.

8. A note on fish. White fish, such as cod, is generally far less fatty than redder fish like kippers or sardines. However, fatty fish are really an excellent source of so many nutrients vital to the pregnant woman, that we feel she should eat them whenever she feels like them. However, they are so rich in nutrients that a small to moderate portion should be enough on any one day.

### Carbohydrates

Carbohydrate may take many forms. It is present in quite a complex form (starch) in many foods, such as cereals and cereal products, potatoes, and in smaller quantities in many other plant foods. Carbohydrate may also occur naturally as simple sugars; for example, fruit sugar or fructose as it is often called, occurs, together with glucose, in many fruits. There is a sugar in milk called lactose. Generally speaking, naturally occurring forms of carbohydrate are desirable because the foods that contain them are also sources of protein, minerals and vitamins. Even diabetics may be able to tolerate carbohydrates as they occur in natural products such as milk and fruit. However, sugar as we buy it in bags is a highly refined product. This type of sugar (sucrose) contains no vitamins, minerals or protein. We eat far too much of it. It is difficult to avoid because sugar is also added to a great many foods. It is present, for example, in cakes, biscuits, lemonade, chocolate, sweets, and even some more savoury products such as tinned peas and baked beans. However, efforts should be made to avoid sugar, by:

1. Cutting down or avoiding biscuits, cakes, sweets, chocolates, jams, ice cream, sweet drinks, fruit tinned in syrup. Many of these products are also very high in fat, so there is a double reason for avoiding them. If you find it impossible to cut such foods out of your diet entirely, do not despair. Keep them to a minimum. For example, you might choose to have a sweet treat just once a day, at a particular time. Or, you might like to bake your own products, using less fat and sugar than the recipe tells you.

2. If your appetite is satisfied with other savoury products, you will feel less inclined to eat sweet things. So, having well-balanced regular meals is very important.

3. If you want a snack, have a savoury food. If you really cannot resist something sweet, try fresh bread with a small quantity of low sugar jam, or a banana sandwich, or fresh fruit chopped into a plain yogurt.

*Fibre*
It is recommended that everyone has much more fibre in their diet. Fibre is the unabsorbed part of the foods we eat, a type of complex carbohydrate found in the cell walls of plants. Fibre helps to keep the gut healthy, working smoothly and efficiently. Obviously, this will be extra important for the expectant mother, because she will have to fight against the tendency to constipation so often associated with pregnancy. There is *no* particular need to buy bags of bran and add large spoonfuls of the stuff to the things you eat! Bran (and other forms of fibre) are readily available in many kinds of food. Here are some examples:

1. wholemeal breakfast cereals, such as Weetabix, Shredded Wheat, porridge oats, muesli (preferably, make up your own; nearly all brands have sugar added)
2. wholemeal flour and wholemeal bread
3. brown rice and brown spaghetti
4. fresh fruit
5. vegetables (especially peas and beans). It's probably best to have either fresh or frozen vegetables because tinned varieties have sugar and/or salt added.
6. dried fruit, such as figs, dates, apricots, prunes.

You can see that the foods which contain fibre have already been recommended earlier in this chapter because they contain very many useful nutrients too! It is wise to have at least one fibre-rich food at each meal.

### Salt

The salt we usually use is a type called sodium chloride. We eat many times the amount our bodies actually need. Excess salt intake has been associated with high blood pressure. Also, the body may tend to retain too much fluid if too much salt is eaten. A high salt intake is partly due to habits established when learning to prepare food. At present you might usually add salt to vegetables when they are cooking, and then add more salt to the food at the table. It is essential to break such habits. Add little, or preferably no salt, when cooking vegetables, rice, spaghetti, or any other dish, *even if* the recipe you are using tells you to add salt. Salt is already present in a great many foods and there is no need to have to add salt to anything. If you absolutely must add something to food, try using only a tiny shake of salt. Or use an alternative type of salt (potassium chloride) available at chemists or health food shops. This type of salt will be known usually by a brand name, such as 'Ruthmol'.

As well as avoiding salt itself, avoid foods with salt obviously with it, like crisps. Processed, smoked or cured meats, such as bacon, are high in salt and so should be strictly limited.

### Summary

Here is a summary of what we've told you so far:
Eat plenty of protein from both animal sources (such as low-fat dairy

products, lean meat, fish) and plant sources (such as bread, rice, spaghetti, cereals, pulses). Have wholegrain cereal products rather than white, refined products whenever possible (for example, have wholemeal bread rather than white).

Eat plenty of fruit and vegetables (especially peas and beans).

*Reduce* fat, sugar (sucrose) and salt intake.

**Planning your meals: some specific examples**
You've been given a great deal of information on nutrition. How are you going to apply this knowledge to planning your daily menu? It's probably best to plan three meals a day. These meals don't all have to be the same size if you don't want them to be. For example, if you like a large evening meal, a small breakfast and an average size lunch, you can keep this combination. However, although the size of the portions of food might vary, each meal, no matter if it is a big meal or a small meal, should ideally contain proteins (try to include proteins from plant sources such as bread or rice, as well as proteins from animal sources) plus vegetables and/or fruit. If you are a person who likes more than three meals a day, have as many meals as you like, maybe four or five or even six, BUT the portions at each meal will have to be very small in order to avoid taking in surplus fuel which will turn to fat! If you only eat once a day, perhaps you might like to rethink your eating habits very slightly. Still have your large main meal, but have a little less than usual. Add one or two *very* small meals to your daily diet. This will help you if you are suffering from feelings of nausea or heartburn. More smaller meals rather than one very large one should help relieve symptoms.

Are you a person who has three main meals, but snacks in between? Now this is perfectly all right provided you plan the snacks as you would a meal. That is, a snack should contain protein foods or vegetables or fruit or some kind of mixture of these three. Examples are, banana sandwich; beans on toast; fresh fruit milkshake, made with no sugar; a slice of wholemeal toast and a glass of milk. What a snack should *not* be is a biscuit or cake or chocolate! Additional snacks will probably be very important if you are suffering from sickness in the first trimester. You might find you feel queasy at odd times in the day, or that your stomach feels very unsettled when you first wake in the morning. You then may not feel like eating a meal, but a small piece of dry toast, or dry crispbread (such as Ryvita) will often settle an uneasy stomach. You may find it useful to carry a few crispbread around with you, to nibble on should you suddenly feel queasy. However, this should only last until about the 13th week of pregnancy, and should, fortunately, be unnecessary after that!

If you find you are putting on too much weight, you are probably eating too large portions at each meal or snack. Cut down very slightly, and be extra rigorous with keeping fat and sugar intake to an absolute minimum. Exercise a little more if you can. It you're not putting on enough pregnancy weight (roughly 1 lb or 0.45 kg a week after the first trimester), then eat slightly larger portions of the foods we recommend. In the examples of breakfasts and main meals that we give you later in this section, we have deliberately not specified exact size of portions in nearly all cases. This is because each woman will have her own needs; some will need to eat more than others in order to put on exactly the right amount of weight. You yourself should adjust the size of the portions to keep your weight gain exactly right for the pregnancy. Do remember though, that we recommend *at least* 1 pint of milk a day; have more if you do not have yogurt or cheese.

*Ideas for meals*
Whenever milk is listed in the menus we are about to give you, use skimmed or semi-skimmed varieties if you can. Vegans might like to have soya milk as they do not drink animal milk. But vegans should take supplements; soya milk may not contain as much calcium as cow's milk. If fruit is listed, this means fresh fruit. Where cereal products are mentioned (such as bread or rice) use wholemeal or wholegrain if possible. If you want butter or margarine, use the smallest amount possible. Try not to use salt at all. If you can't do without sugar in a meal (for example, on breakfast cereal), limit yourself to one very small spoonful. If you really like jam or marmalade on bread or toast, and cannot do without, use only one tiny spoonful, preferably of a low sugar variety.

## BREAKFASTS

1. Shredded Wheat, milk, fruit
2. Weetabix, milk, fruit
3. muesli, milk, fruit
4. a bran type cereal, such as 'All-bran' or 'Branflakes', milk, fruit
5. yogurt (plain) with fresh or dried, chopped fruit, nuts, and perhaps a little wheatgerm mixed in.
6. porridge oats, milk, fruit
7. soak some dried apricots, dried prunes, or other dried fruit overnight. Have these with any kind of wholegrain cereal (especially nice with muesli). Add plain yogurt or milk.
8. kipper, bread, fruit, glass milk
9. sardines or pilchards on toast, tomato, glass milk
10. one egg, toast, fruit or tomato, glass milk
11. cheese and tomatoes on toast
12. welsh rarebit on toast, tomato
13. beans on toast, glass milk, fruit
14. two small, well-grilled rashers of bacon, tomato, bread, glass milk
15. toast, fruit, glass milk
16. dried fruit and nuts. Have some fresh fruit as well if you like, and a glass of milk
17. lean meat or fish of any kind, bread, glass milk, fruit
18. milk shake made with fresh fruit, milk, *no* sugar. Add an egg if you like, or perhaps a little wheatgerm.

Remember, portions do not need to be enormous in order for you to feel satisfied. If, by any chance, you finish your chosen breakfast and you still feel hungry, you can always have a slice of toast in addition.

The breakfasts listed here are to give you a basic idea of what to eat. Feel free to pursue your own ideas, provided they follow the nutritional guidelines we have already laid out.

Try to eat enough at breakfast to keep you satisfied until lunchtime. You shouldn't need to snack on foods in the morning, except, perhaps, if you are suffering from early pregnancy sickness. If you suddenly start to feel queasy, nibble on toast or crispbread. If you feel sick before breakfast, slowly eat a piece of dry toast or crispbread *before* getting out of bed. Either get someone else to bring this to you, or take it to bed with you the night before.

## MAIN MEALS

*Meat meals*
1. liver and onions, peas, carrots, potatoes, glass milk
2. portion of any lean meat, jacket or boiled potato, peas or beans, one other vegetable, glass milk
3. corned beef sandwiches with a tomato, plain yogurt or glass milk
4. lean meat, salad (include sweetcorn or peas or beans), potatoes or bread, glass milk. (Make up a meat and salad sandwich with the ingredients if you like.)
5. meat and vegetable curry and rice. Use only a little meat (around 2 oz (56 gm) per person). Include pulses (peas or beans or lentils) with the vegetables. Have a glass of milk or add plain yogurt to the curry. Fruit can either be eaten after the main course, or used as an ingredient in the curry.
6. lasagne (use only a little meat and supplement with soya meat or lentils), salad, glass milk
7. cottage pie. Use less meat than you normally would and add either soya meat, lentils or peas to the mix. Eat with carrots or a salad. You can either top the cottage pie with grated cheese or have a glass of milk with the meal.
8. meat and vegetable casserole or stew. Use only a small amount of lean meat. Add milk to the liquid the vegetables and meat are in, or have a glass of milk separately
9. spaghetti bolognese. Again, supplement the meat with soya meat or lentils so that you need to use less animal meat. Have a glass of milk or, alternatively, top the meal with a little grated cheese. Finish with a piece of fruit
10. chilli con carne and rice, and a salad. Use only a little meat but use plenty of red beans. Finish with a glass of milk

*Fish meals*
1. prawn or salmon sandwiches, glass milk, fruit
2. sardines or pilchards or toast, glass milk, fruit
3. fish pie. Top the pie with grated cheese and tomato. Eat the

pie with carrots and peas, or a salad
4. fish fingers, baked beans or peas, potato, glass milk
5. a portion of fish (preferably not fried), potatoes (either boiled, baked in their skins, or fried as very thick cut chips), peas. If you've bought your meal from the chip shop and you want to keep the fat content down, leave some of the batter from the fish, and do not eat the smaller, thinner chips
6. cold fish (such as salmon or prawns) with a salad, bread or potatoes, glass of milk
7. a portion of white fish, broccoli or spinach, a little grated cheese, tomato
8. a portion of 'oily' red fish (such as kippers, mackerel, sardines), bread, tomato, glass milk
9. haddock with a poached egg on top, peas, glass milk
10. prawn curry, rice, peas, glass milk

*Egg/cheese meals*
Eggs and cheese are both high in fat. It is unadvisable, therefore, to have very large portions of these foods.

1. egg or cheese sandwiches. Include some salad (like a tomato) in the sandwiches
2. cheese and tomato on toast
3. cheese and potato pie, peas or a green leafy vegetable, carrots
4. egg and/or cheese salad (include pulses with the salad), bread or potatoes or rice or pasta (some of these can be used in the salad)
5. broccoli or spinach or leeks or cauliflower, with a cheese sauce, one other vegetable
6. a two-egg omelette, mushrooms, peas, tomatoes (the vegetables can be a part of the omelette, if liked), glass milk
7. jacket potato, grated cheese or an egg, tomato, sweetcorn or peas
8. pizza (try making your own with a wholemeal flour base, made with only a little fat)
9. lentil or vegetable soup, topped with a little grated cheese, bread, fruit
10. one scrambled egg, toast, glass milk, fruit

*Meals with no protein from animal sources*
You can, of course, add protein from an animal source very simply
to any of these meals, by drinking a glass of milk with them.
Vegans (who consume no animal produce) would do well to drink
a fortified soya milk with each meal instead.

1. Use soya beans (or soya meat, a derivative of the soya bean) to
   make any of the meals listed under meat meals. Soya, although
   not nutritionally identical to meat, is a very good substitute for
   meat. Soya beans or soya meat (available from health food
   shops, some chemists, some supermarkets) can be used to
   make, for example, curries, chilli con carne, lasagne (use pasta
   without egg in it). spaghetti bolognese, stuffed marrow,
   cottage pie, wholemeal pitta bread stuffed with a vegetable
   and soya mixture. Soya meat can be a bit bland if you are
   unused to it, so be generous in your use of spices. Dehydrated
   soya meat, instead of being soaked in boiling water, can be
   soaked in Bisto gravy (surprisingly, a vegan product) to give
   it more flavour. Alternatively, tomato juice can be used to
   give flavour; soya mince can be added for five minutes or so to
   heated tomato juice or tinned tomatoes. Some soya meats are
   enriched with $B_{12}$, a very necessary additive for vegans. Have
   fruit, salad or vegetables, with any of the meals you make with
   soya meat.
2. sliced banana on toast. Sprinkle with chopped nuts and sultanas
3. baked beans on toast, fruit
4. fruit crumble. Slice apples (or any fresh fruit you fancy), and
   add sultanas and a few flaked almonds. Cover with a crumble
   made from wholemeal flour plus a small amount of soya flour,
   with a little vegan margarine rubbed in. Use half or quarter
   the amount of fat you would usually use for pastry. Add no
   sugar.
5. 3oz (84gm) sultanas, 2oz (56gm) almonds or brazils, fruit
6. jacket potato or bread, salad (include pulses), nuts, fruit
7. lentil or pea soup, bread, nuts, fruit
8. vegetable curry and rice, fruit
9. pancakes made from wholemeal flour, soya flour, and a little
   fat. Add fruit (such as chopped apple, banana, sultanas) and
   nuts (such as flaked almonds) to the pancake. Use no sugar.

10. rice pudding made with brown rice, soya milk, and sultanas. Add no sugar.

You should now have a very good idea of what nutritionally well-balanced meals look like. Naturally, we hope that many or all of the foods we have mentioned will be familiar to you. We have deliberately tried to be very practical in our examples of meals you might like to eat. If we had listed very exotic or difficult recipes for meals, you would be less likely to follow and use them. However, *do* experiment with your own recipes, using the nutritional advice that we have given you. There are now many excellent recipe books available to give you ideas on low fat meals, high fibre meals, etc.

We would like to stress that although we have recommended a healthy, nutritious eating pattern, with lower fat, sugar and salt than you are probably used to, we do realize that you might find it difficult to follow such a regime to begin with. So, make the changes gradually and slowly if you cannot do them all at once. Just cut down on the undesirable products to begin with if you feel you simply wouldn't like life without them. And, of course, to a certain extent such products are traditional at various times. We have pancakes on pancake day (Shrove Tuesday), Christmas pudding and Christmas cake, chocolate Easter eggs, gifts of confectionery at birthdays, and so on. We are not asking that you totally do without these things, especially if it's going to make you feel miserable or deprived. You are only likely to respond to such a feeling by having an enormous binge of the 'forbidden' foods at some time or another. Rather, you should limit your consumption of these foods so that you do not feel deprived, but at the same time, you are not ruining your health by eating them excessively. For example, if it is Christmas, and there is cake or pudding at the end of the meal, and you want some, then have it. However, bear in mind that if you really want to enjoy it, you should still be a little hungry after the main course, so do not eat *quite* as much of this as you normally might. A golden rule is never to eat if you are not hungry. If you find your portion of food is too large, don't be afraid to leave it. This especially applies to foods like Christmas cake or Christmas pudding. It is very easy to misjudge, cut yourself a medium portion, but then find, halfway through, that it's too much. Never force yourself to eat. Try to be aware of feelings of fullness that tell you when you have had enough. Try to eat slowly and don't hurry your meals.

If you've been given chocolates, or if you have something like sweets or biscuits in the house, plan when you are going to eat these foods, in the same way that you plan meals. If you find that you cannot do without these foods completely, think about when it is best to eat them. Choose a specific time of day (for example, at the end of dinner) when you will have a small sweet thing. Enjoy it as a part of the meal, but try to limit your sweet treat to this. This is much better than absent-mindedly nibbling sweets or biscuits or chocolate all through the day. You can consume far too much of the wrong foods this way, and it is also far worse for the teeth.

Think about which pattern of eating suits you best. Let us say you decide on three meals plus two snacks each day. Plan these events in so far as you can. Make them nutritionally sound, with protein foods, fruit and/or vegetables. However, if you really want a sweet treat, limit it to once a day at maximum, if you can. Think about where you are going to eat your meals or snacks. Don't just grab food whilst doing other things. Concentrate on your food. Think about what it tastes like whilst you are eating it. Try not to eat between the meal and snack times you have planned. You should feel hungry, and really ready to eat, at the start of each meal or snack. Eat until satisfied, then stop.

This may all sound very obvious, but very many people, with difficulties with weight control, do not do these things. They might nibble at food almost constantly during the day. They never approach a meal feeling properly hungry. They eat all that is on the plate because it is there, rather than stopping when they feel full. Watching television is also a very common prompt to eat. Many people with obesity problems find they consume large quantities of food, without even thinking about it, whilst watching television each evening. Such habits must be broken. It is much easier to break them if you concentrate instead on positive aspects of health, good meal planning, and more exercise as part of everyday life. Include the rest of your family in your plans if you can. Nearly everyone would benefit from being more active, and from eating a diet lower in fat, sugar and salt, and higher in fibre-rich foods.

## Morning sickness (pregnancy nausea), food cravings, and heartburn

These ailments are all often associated with pregnancy. We have already mentioned them in passing, but because nearly every pregnant woman experiences them to some extent, a little extra advice is called for:

*Morning sickness (pregnancy nausea)*
A feeling of slight sickness is very common during the first trimester, although most women are not *actually* sick very often. Such unpleasant side effects may occur in the morning (hence, morning sickness) or, in fact, at any time of the day. With some women, they do not occur at all.

To stop, or at least to minimize these feelings of sickness, avoid very fatty food, or sweet or spicy foods. Eat small, frequent meals, planned as we have shown you. Carry dry toast or crispbreads with you, and *slowly* eat a *little* of this food if you are suddenly overcome with feelings of nausea. Have some dry toast or crispbread when you awake in the morning, before you get out of bed.

You will almost certainly find that you develop a strong dislike for certain foods, even foods you really liked before you became pregnant. Examples are fried foods, fatty foods generally, sweet foods and confectionery. You may feel repulsed by coffee, strong tea, and alcohol. Sometimes, just the smell of such foods or drinks will make you feel sick, so be extra careful to avoid them.

Some women start to dislike sound, nutritious foods or drinks. For instance, many women find a drink of milk brings on waves of nausea. However, ordinary milk is very fatty, and the answer could well be to switch to skimmed or semi-skimmed milk. Alternatively, have cheese or plain yogurt to satisfy your need for calcium. Acidic fruits like grapefruits or oranges, or soft, sweet fruits like plums or strawberries may be upsetting to the stomach. Don't let it worry you. Either pick a less sweet tasting or acidic fruit (you might still like apples, for instance), or alternatively, increase the amount of vegetables and salad foods that you eat. No one particular food is essential. If you go off a food, try to pick an acceptable alternative to supply you with the nutrients you need.

*Food cravings*

Although you will probably start to dislike foods you previously enjoyed, this does not mean you will lose your appetite entirely. You may well experience a very strong desire for certain foods, perhaps types that you never much liked before you were pregnant. You might, for example, suddenly find you crave large portions of meat or fish, even if you didn't much like these foods before. If you crave any type of food we have mentioned as good, nutritious and beneficial, in our review of food earlier in this chapter, then eat it until your appetite is satisfied. Have as much protein from animal and plant sources, vegetables and fruit, as you desire. Do be careful here though. It is very easy to overestimate the amount of food you need to satisfy a craving. You may well feel, at the beginning of a meal, that only an enormous steak will satisfy your craving for meat. Half-way through you may discover, though, that you've had enough. Never feel guilty about not eating all the food you've prepared. It will usually keep for another occasion. Or give the dog a treat.

What if you crave a food high in sugar or fat, such as cakes, biscuits or sweets? Don't indulge such a craving if you can help it. If you eat sugary foods, you will get an almost immediate feeling of relief, as your blood sugar level quickly rises. Unfortunately, however, the body then overcompensates for this quick rise in blood sugar level, and the result is that blood sugar falls to a level *below* the one it was at before you started eating. You then feel very hungry indeed, and the temptation is to eat more sugary food. This is a vicious circle, and can lead to you eating a great deal of food, more than you need, and as a result you become fat. Sweet foods are not going to supply you with as many of the essential nutrients as the other kinds of foods we've mentioned earlier, all the types of protein foods, vegetables and fruits. If you're having sensible, planned meals based on these foods, and are eating until you are satisfied, you shouldn't crave foods high in sugar or fat. If you do, it could be a sign you are not eating enough at meals. So, if you crave sugary and fatty foods, first try eating something more acceptable. Plan a snack or meal, as we have shown you, from foods high in essential nutrients. If you still yearn, say, for a biscuit or a cream bun after you have eaten your snack or meal, do not rush to the nearest shop and buy up all available stocks. Instead, plan a treat to include a little of this food. Have a *small* portion of this food as a *part* of the next meal. But don't give into such cravings too often, or you might well put on surplus fat.

*Heartburn*
Heartburn is the sensation of the acidic contents of the stomach travelling back up into the food pipe, and creating a burning sensation. This is especially likely in pregnancy, as hormones act to relax the muscular valve at the upper part of the stomach, allowing food to travel back up. The end of the pregnancy might also be a difficult time, as the enlarged womb presses up against the stomach.

To help avoid heartburn, don't have heavy meals. Avoid spicy foods. Have more frequent, light meals, low in fat and sugar. Don't lie down flat after a meal. If you feel you really want to lie down, prop up the top part of your body with pillows or cushions, hence making it less easy for the food in the stomach to travel back upwards. Ask your doctor for some special preparation or tablets if you like, but it's generally best to try to control heartburn and other ailments associated with pregnancy by controlling your food intake in the ways we have recommended.

# 5

# Exercise and Pregnancy

**Effects of exercise**

Historically speaking, it is only fairly recently that pregnancy has become so intimately involved with medicine. This involvement has undoubtedly done a great deal to save the lives of many mothers and babies, and to improve the health and well-being of even more. An unfortunate effect of the association of pregnancy and medicine, however, is that to many people pregnancy is now almost regarded as some kind of illness. People talk of the 'symptoms' of pregnancy but this does not mean that the pregnant woman is incapable of any kind of effort or exertion without harming herself or the baby. In fact, pregnancy is, of course, a perfectly natural state for a woman. The pregnant woman is usually a healthy woman, and often capable of a great deal more activity than is generally supposed. As far as the baby is concerned, physical activity on the part of the mother is extremely unlikely to decrease its chances of survival. Packed safely in its bag of amniotic fluid, for most of the pregnancy it remains cushioned from the physical jolts and knocks which the mother may encounter. In the days before safe legal abortion was available, women who wished to terminate their pregnancy would often perform horrendous acts, such as jumping down a flight of stairs in an attempt to induce abortion. Typically, the consequence of such acts would be severe injury for the woman, with no harm coming to the baby.

On the other hand, as we have seen in earlier chapters, pregnancy does produce a number of changes in a woman's body and it is important that we pay attention to these when we come to consider the role of exercise in pregnancy. It is also important to recognize that there are different types of exercise, with different effects on the body. In deciding on suitable exercise for the pregnant woman, therefore, we need to look both at what the woman is capable of, and what benefits the exercise is required to provide.

To most people exercise involves some uncomfortable, often boring, physical effort which they would rather avoid if possible. However, it is now widely recognized that exercise is not only beneficial but that it is actually essential for good health. As one doctor pointed out recently, we are often advised to see our GPs if we intend to take up exercise after the age of 30, but it may be even more important to see the GP if we intend NOT to exercise after the age of 30. We are often told that exercise can be dangerous, but it is worth remembering that failure to exercise may be even more dangerous.

Regular exercise has a number of effects on the body. Exactly what effect it has will depend on the kind of exercise, how intensely and regularly it is performed and so on. Three of the main effects exercise can have are increasing *Strength*, increasing *Stamina* and increasing *Suppleness* – the three S's of physical fitness. It is important to consider each of these when looking at the place of exercise in a healthy pregnancy.

At first glance *Strength* might seem to be of minor importance to many women, who may regard themselves as being as strong as they wish to be, and who may fear developing large muscles. However, increased strength may be of great value in pregnancy. For example, as we saw in Chapter 2, backache is not unusual in pregnant women. Suitable exercises to strengthen the relevant body muscles can enable a woman to avoid the risk of backache.

Increased *Stamina* is perhaps closest to what we normally think of when we talk of being physically fit. By increased stamina we do not mean any particular increase in strength of the body, but rather an increase in its endurance. Increasing stamina may not enable you to perform feats of strength of which you were previously incapable, but the things you do will not tire you so much, and you will be able to continue your activities for longer. So, for example, increased stamina associated with the leg muscles may not make you run any faster, but it will enable you to run farther. The kind of exercise which increases stamina is of particular importance to us here, because it is this kind of exercise which has most influence on weight control.

When we come to *Suppleness*, the situation is rather different, since pregnancy itself will automatically make a woman more supple. As we saw in Chapter 2, the hormonal changes in a woman's body will tend to soften the tissue of which tendons and ligaments are made. This enables joints to move over a greater range than previously, something which is essential, for example, during birth when joints in the hip bones need to extend sufficiently for the baby to pass through. Unfortunately, this softening of the tendons and ligaments also presents problems. Joints may become weaker because bones are no longer being held so tightly together. As a result, the wrong kind of exercise may lead to damage.

## Types of exercise; aerobic or anaerobic?

Looked at in detail, there are obviously hundreds if not thousands of different kinds of exercise. Taken more broadly, however, these may be divided into a few general categories. Some, for example, are part of competitive games like squash, netball etc., whilst others are simply routines in themselves, like yoga, dance classes etc. One of the most important distinctions in the field of exercise is between those exercises which are aerobic and those which are anaerobic. We can see the difference when we compare, say, running flat out and walking at a comfortable pace. In the first case most people would soon be out of breath and have to stop; in the second, most people would be able to continue for some length of time without having to stop or even noticing any change in their breathing. All forms of exercise use energy. The difference between aerobic and anaerobic exercise lies in the rate at which the energy is used. When using energy the body demands oxygen, which we supply by breathing in and out. If we are only using energy very slowly, as in walking, it is easy to keep up with the body's demands for oxygen by breathing perhaps a little more deeply or a little more rapidly. This is aerobic exercise. As the energy is used up faster, however, for example when running flat out, the demand for oxygen becomes so great that no matter how fast or deeply we breathe, we can't supply the body with as much oxygen as it requires. When this happens the body starts to use a different process to produce energy, one which is less efficient but which needs less oxygen. This is anaerobic exercise. This reduced efficiency of anaerobic exercise means that the body is unable to continue the exercise for as long. We can see this effect when we compare how long we continue walking at an even pace and for how short a time we can run flat out.

During pregnancy, and indeed before and after, most of the useful exercise will be aerobic, that is to say, it won't involve getting completely out of breath. For most women, the kind of violent exercise which produces total breathlessness will not be appropriate during pregnancy. Exercises such as gentle cycling or swimming, jogging, walking and so on may be chosen, although some may need more care than others. Any form of exercise will involve some risk, although this will usually be small and for most people the risk associated with not exercising will be much higher. In order to decide on the right type of exercise, therefore, it is useful to look at some of the possible dangers.

### General dangers of exercise

From time to time the TV, newspapers and the like report horror stories of the 'dangers' of exercise; a runner having a heart attack in a race, swimmers suffering attacks of cramp and nearly drowning, and so on. It is certainly true that some forms of exercise and sport are dangerous. Injuries, and even death, are not unknown in sports such as hang-gliding, boxing and rugby for example. It is probably a safe bet, however, that these are not the sports likely to be taken up by a pregnant woman. Even 'safe' sports and exercises can be dangerous if started and continued without some degree of care. The pregnant woman, whose body is undergoing a number of unfamiliar changes, will need to be a little more cautious than most people if harm or injury is to be avoided. Fortunately, the risks are few, and the precautions necessary are largely quite simple, and often a matter of common sense and a little knowledge. For total safety, it is obviously necessary to know what the general risks are, and what special considerations apply during pregnancy.

In understanding the general risks of exercise, it is helpful to know a little bit about what happens in the body during exercise.

Practically all forms of exercise will affect all of the three Ss – *Strength, Stamina* and *Suppleness*. However, each of the three will not be affected equally. For most people, for example, slow gentle swimming will only have a slight effect on suppleness, with perhaps a little more effect on strength; most of the benefit will be in terms of increased stamina. A yoga class on the other hand may have only a slight effect on stamina but will considerably increase suppleness.

All exercise involves making higher demands on the body than those to which it is accustomed. Safe exercising is simply a matter of making sure that the demands are not too much higher than the body is normally used to. One of the most obvious lessons to learn from this is that any exercise should be taken up gradually, increasing the demands on the body bit by bit as it becomes capable of more and more. For most people this is relatively straightforward, although for a tiny minority the increase will have to be EXTREMELY gradual, and the upper limit of the body's capabilities may be quite low, meaning that even after training there is a limit to what the individual can manage. Fortunately, the human body is equipped with a remarkably good system for warning us when we are putting ourselves at risk – the feeling of pain. Forget completely the old motto that 'if it hurts it must be doing you good' – this may apply to top level Olympic athletes, but as far as simple exercises for health is concerned it is just WRONG. A feeling of pain is the body's way of warning you that it is at risk of harm, and that you may be overdoing things. Continuing to push yourself too hard may lead to injury or other harm; placing the body under continual stress may also result in it being less capable of fighting off infections, and thus lead to illness – exactly the opposite of what you're trying to achieve.

One of the biggest fears for most people taking up exercise is that their heart will be unable to cope. Stories of people suffering heart attacks during exercise appear in the newspapers from time to time, giving comfort to those who are looking for an excuse not to bother exercising. Certainly, most forms of exercise will involve at least a little extra demand on the heart; many forms will require the heart to work considerably harder than normal. In a person whose heart is already working close to its limits, any extra demand may be dangerous.

Fortunately, few women of child-bearing age are likely to be at extreme risk of heart failure. For a start, women are less susceptible to heart attacks than men. Moreover, most women who are pregnant or about to become pregnant are likely to be quite young; few will be over 40 years of age. Again, younger people are less likely to suffer heart attacks than older people.

Some of the general cautions about taking exercise which apply to the general population will, however, also apply to young women. In particular, women who are very overweight and who are heavy smokers should be careful about starting to exercise. Women who have taken the contraceptive pill for a long period of time, particularly if they are over 30, should also be careful. In Chapter 8 we will look at some of the ways in which you can make a rough assessment of your present state of fitness; if there is any reason to suspect you may be at risk of heart problems (for example, if you have one or more parents with heart problems) you should consult your own doctor before trying anything at all strenuous or difficult. For most women doing gentle exercise, however, the risk of heart problems is very low indeed, whether pregnant or not.

As far as most of us are concerned, however, the dangers of exercise are rather less serious than possible heart attacks. Many of the risks are specific to the form of exercise undertaken, whilst others may be a result of several types of exercise. If well taught by an experienced instructor, most forms of exercise are usually quite safe, although it is still important to remember not to force the body to do things which are uncomfortable or painful.

A type of problem which may affect people who start an exercise programme over-enthusiastically is the 'overuse injury'. This type of injury, as its name suggests, results from using some part of the body excessively. For example, a person who takes up jogging may be overkeen in the early stages and run too far, too soon. A bone like the shin bone is thus subjected to a quite unaccustomed and repetitive pounding and eventually may crack or break altogether – an injury known as a stress fracture. Such injuries may also occur in trained athletes, particularly if they attempt a sudden increase in the amount of their training. Once again, the answer is to avoid anything which produces pain or discomfort. Do not assume that such a problem couldn't happen to you because you aren't doing enough to cause any harm. At least one physiotherapist specializing in sports injuries has reported a case of a woman having the beginnings of a stress fracture on her third day of jogging, having done 1 minute on her first day, 2 minutes on her second and 3 on her third. Fortunately, most of us are nowhere near so fragile and simply reducing the level of exercise slightly when pain occurs will enable us to maintain a healthy level of activity without injury. Of course, if pain persists, or if even the slightest level of exercise is painful, you should consult your doctor for advice.

Like heart attacks, serious injuries like stress fractures are uncommon and the majority of people taking up exercise will do so without any serious problems. Much more common are a number of minor problems such as muscular aches, sprains, bruises and so on. Many of these can be avoided by adopting a sensible and careful approach to exercise. Part of being sensible and careful involves not only recognizing the risks we have just discussed but also of recognizing that the state of pregnancy itself introduces certain complications and additional risks to exercise.

### Exercise risks associated with pregnancy

Perhaps one of the major worries that any woman has is of damaging or even losing her baby if she exercises during pregnancy. For a variety of medical reasons, some women will find it difficult to carry a baby to term. Some women tend to miscarry, and it is usually advised that such women rest as much as possible in order to avoid losing their baby. If your doctor advises rest you must do so. However, we cannot emphasize too strongly that if you are a fit and healthy young woman, then in all probability you will be able to remain physically active throughout your pregnancy.

There are, however, a number of less serious risks associated with exercise in pregnancy. We saw in Chapter 2 how the hormone progesterone produces a softening of the body's ligaments and tendons in order to prepare for birth. During this period there may be additional risks from certain types of exercise. For example, if your exercise puts too much strain on the feet, the joints may become realigned causing 'flat feet'. Not only is the development of flat feet potentially very painful, it is also likely to cause problems in the future. The arches of the feet serve an important function in providing flexibility and support, and if the arches fall, the woman may be more at risk of other injuries associated with such activities as walking and running. This does not mean that you cannot run and walk during pregnancy, but does mean that good supportive footwear is essential. For both ordinary walking and running, conventional runners' training shoes are excellent, providing a useful combination of cushioning and support. If buying such shoes, it is worth going to a specialist running shop and spending some time over your choice. Ask the advice of the sales staff, and try several pairs of shoes until you find a pair that is comfortable. Shop late in the day rather than early; your feet are smaller in the mornings and a pair which seem like a good fit in the early morning may prove to be much too tight during exercise, when your feet will swell. By the end of the afternoon your feet will have swollen to about the size they will be during exercise, and you are more likely to obtain a pair of suitable size. Pregnancy itself, of course, may lead to a swelling of feet and ankles; however, if you follow the advice on diet in this book, such swelling will be minimal or non-existent.

The stretching of tendons and ligaments also suggests that you should be careful about exercises like dance and yoga which place a high demand on suppleness. Whilst it may be tempting to make the most of the increase in suppleness during pregnancy, it is important that the development of the muscles, to which the tendons are attached, keeps pace with any extra suppleness. You will need to be especially careful about the muscles in your back. The individual bones (verbebrae) which make your spine rely a great deal on having the right muscular support to maintain their structure. The softening of tendons means that the muscles have to work a little bit harder to keep the vertebrae properly positioned, and the softening of ligaments means that the vertebrae are less effectively held together. This does not mean that you should avoid exercising these muscles during pregnancy; indeed, since it is important that these muscles be capable of coping with the extra demands, pregnancy may be a time when exercise is especially important. Remember, though, that for exercise to be beneficial it needs to be combined with REST. Keeping the right combination of exercise and rest will enable you to maintain good health and to avoid the various kinds of back pain from which so many people suffer. Softening of tissue does not mean that exercise is not possible during pregnancy, but merely that a little common sense and care is needed. As always, recognize that pain is a sign of trying too hard, and means it is time to ease off a little. With sense and care, most women will be able to exercise without any problem; any persistent pain, particularly in your feet, knees or back should, of course, be reported to your doctor.

An aspect of exercise which may give much cause for concern is its effect on your blood pressure. During most forms of exercise the body is going to require an increase in the blood supply to the muscles concerned. Remember that even during aerobic exercise the body will be demanding more oxygen; once this oxygen has been taken in by breathing, it needs to be transported to the muscles which need it. This transportation is done by the red blood cells. Any reasonable increase in demand for oxygen will mean that the red cells have to travel faster round the body, picking up oxygen in the lungs and depositing it at the muscles which need it. At the same time the muscles which are working will be producing waste products which need to be taken away. For all this to happen, the red cells have to be pushed faster around the body – which is why your heart beats faster when you are exercising. Remember, too, that the heart is itself a muscle; by having to beat faster it, too, will need to increase its own blood supply. The outcome of all this is that the heart pushes the blood harder and harder in order to move it faster around the body. Because it is pushing harder, the pressure in the arteries rises, since more has to be pushed through much the same amount of space in any period of time. It's rather like trying to get lots of people through a narrow doorway; if you let them go through slowly, at their own pace, there need be no particular pressure. If, however, you try to push everyone through very quickly, they will end up being squeezed together. Most problematic as far as the body is concerned, is that not only would the people press harder and harder against each other, but they would also press harder against the side of the doorway. Similarly, in the blood supply an increase in pressure within veins and arteries means that there is increasing pressure on the walls of these blood vessels. If at any point there is a weakness in one of these, the extra pressure can cause the blood vessel to burst, with potentially serious consequences. If the blood vessel is in the brain, for example, such a burst will result in a stroke.

Obviously, the increase in blood pressure caused by exercise is usually no more than the body can cope with, since most people who exercise suffer no ill effects. However, those with unduly high blood pressure to start with may be at risk. Pregnancy may produce its own changes in blood pressure, but these are usually relatively small compared to the short-term changes which exercise may produce. For most women, pregnancy is more likely to produce a reduction in blood pressure during the middle trimester, with normal blood pressure during the first and third trimesters. In some women, especially those with an initially high blood pressure, pregnancy may produce a rise in blood pressure which can lead to a condition called pre-eclampsia (discussed in Chapter 2). Women with pre-eclampsia, or pre-eclampsic toxaemia as it is sometimes called, should NOT attempt to exercise during pregnancy but should carefully follow their doctor's advice regarding rest. In a few women blood pressure may rise above normal at the end of pregnancy or remain at a higher level for some time following the birth. Again, such women should be careful about exercising at such times.

Fortunately, all pregnant women will have their blood pressure checked regularly at ante-natal clinics, so any danger signs here will be immediately apparent. Whilst measurement of blood pressure is not always totally accurate, the obtained measurements are more likely to be overestimates than underestimates, that is to say they will be on 'the safe side'. For example, if you are in a hurry to reach the clinic, this may have the effect of temporarily pushing your blood pressure up to some degree, and when measured, it might appear that your blood pressure is higher than it should be. Obviously, such a rise is only brief and is not really anything to worry about. Often, if your doctor thinks this is what has happened, you will be asked to sit and rest for a short while after which the first reading will be checked. There are a few things which can produce a temporary drop in blood pressure, but for most of these, the effect is so short that it would not affect the measurement in the clinic.

Of course, not all kinds of exercise produce the same changes in blood pressure, and it is important to distinguish between the long-term and short-term effects of exercise. Some forms of exercise, for example, may produce a temporary increase in blood pressure, but if the exercise is continued for several weeks or months, the person's normal blood pressure may become lower. The amount of increase in blood pressure in the short-term is not simply a matter of how hard or prolonged the exercise is. Isometric exercises, for example, where muscles are tensed by pushing or pulling one muscle against another or against an immovable object, have been used by a number of athletes. A typical exercise might involve clasping the hands behind the neck and pulling them forward at the same time pushing the head back; or the person might be required to press hard against a brick wall for a number of seconds. The essential feature of such exercises is that they involve effort without movement; unfortunately, they are also likely to produce very dramatic (although very brief) rises in blood pressure which may be dangerous for some people. Since for most people the main effect of isometric exercises is to produce a fairly rapid gain in muscle bulk, it is likely to be of little value except in body-building. In terms of improving general health care for pregnant women, such exercise has little to recommend it.

Whilst other forms of exercise will not produce such dramatic increases in blood pressure as isometrics, most will bring about some rise. In the vast majority of cases, where blood pressure is normal to start with, this is nothing to worry about. Women who are substantially overweight or whose blood pressure is found to be raised at the ante-natal clinic should, of course, seek their doctor's advice before attempting anything particularly strenuous.

## General benefits of exercise
Surprising as it may seem after all this talk of the risks and dangers of exercise, we still believe that exercise is a good thing for most women during pregnancy. The fact is that with a little bit of caution and common sense, most of the risks associated with exercise can be avoided quite easily. On the other hand, avoiding the risks of NOT exercising can be remarkably difficult.

To many people it may come as a surprise that any exercise at all is recommended in pregnancy. Yet for the majority of women, exercise during pregnancy will present little difficulty. Even the extreme level of exercise performed by successful athletes can be maintained well into pregnancy. The Norwegian Olympic marathon runner Ingrid Kristiansen surprised many people by announcing that she had competed at international level, quite successfully, whilst several months pregnant. A study of several Eastern European athletes who continued to compete during pregnancy found no evidence of harmful consequences from continuing to compete during the first trimester; when they did stop competing, this was because they did not perform quite so well, rather than from any harmful effects. On the other hand, it must be remembered that these were women with several years' training behind them; it would be most unwise for the average woman to attempt a similar level of exercise at any time, pregnant or not.

For the non-athlete, as well as the athlete, however, there is general agreement that exercise may be of considerable benefit during pregnancy. Even 50 years ago a medical encyclopaedia was able to remark that, for the pregnant woman, open air exercise was necessary if at all possible. Amongst the conclusions of a 1976 DHSS study on the effects of exercise were a number relating to pregnancy. Exercise, the authors remarked, is of benefit to pregnant women and '. . . important right up to the end of the pregnancy . . .'. Indeed, not only may exercise make pregnancy more enjoyable and comfortable for the mother, there is considerable evidence to suggest a number of positive health benefits for both mother and baby. Some of these potential benefits are worth looking at more closely.

Just as certain of the risks of exercise apply to most of us, pregnant or not, so do certain of the benefits. Earlier in the chapter we noted that, in general, exercise affects the three Ss – *Strength Stamina* and *Suppleness*. The important thing, of course, is how changes in each of these may be of benefit to us.

One of the first things to note about exercise, and something which may seem a little strange at first, is that many of the benefits relate to the kinds of risks we were talking about earlier. For example, whilst people may worry about the risks of having a heart attack whilst exercising, it is important to remember that people who exercise regularly will usually be less at risk of heart disease than people who do not. Practically all forms of exercise make the heart work harder than normal. As long as the extra work is not too much for the heart to cope with at the time, the heart will gradually come to adapt to the extra demands which you place on it. One of the effects of regular exercise, of practically all forms, is to increase the size and capacity of the heart. This is not something to be frightened of; indeed it can become a life-saver. For a start, if your heart is bigger, it means that it can push more blood round your body with each stroke. Looked at another way, this is the same as saying that to push blood round at a certain rate it doesn't have to beat so fast, that is, it doesn't have to work so hard. Since we've already noted that physical exertion calls for the blood to be pumped round faster, a bigger heart means that the extra demand for blood can be met without making the heart work much harder and certainly making it more likely to be able to cope with whatever physical demands are being made. Moreover, exercise can reduce the risk of heart attacks in other ways. Regular exercise increases the ability of the blood to carry oxygen around the body; again, this means that to supply the body's tissues with the oxygen they need, the heart doesn't have to work so hard. Some of these effects can be quite substantial; the amount of blood the heart pumps each beat can commonly increase 50 per cent or more, and an increase of up to 100 per cent is not rare. To some extent this can be seen by comparing the pulse rates of people who exercise regularly with those who do not. In non-exercising individuals the pulse rate will typically average 70 to 80 beats per minute or more; in a trained athlete the figure may be below 40, meaning that over the same period of time the non-athlete's heart has had to do twice as much work. Finally, it is worth noting that exercise improves the effectiveness with which oxygen in the blood is supplied to the muscles. Since the heart is itself a muscle, this means that it is itself supplied with oxygen; one effect of this is that it is more able to survive any problems which do occur – a blood clot in a cardiac vessel which would stop a normal heart may leave the trained heart with quite sufficient capacity to continue functioning.

In the long term, then, regular exercise can do a great deal to reduce the risk of heart problems. A similar benefit may be apparent with respect to blood pressure, and many experts believe that carefully supervised aerobic exercise may be of help to sufferers from high blood pressure. Whilst it can be difficult to be certain that it is in fact the exercise (rather than some other simultaneous change in lifestyle) which is responsible, it at least suggests the possibility of a further advantage to exercising regularly. Since blood pressure is also affected by the kinds of food we eat (especially by salt intake), this means that considerable relief from the problems of high blood pressure can be possible by following the advice we give in this book.

Finally, it is worth noting that even the minor risks of exercise like sprains, muscular stiffness and the like can be alleviated by regular training. Muscular stiffness is a direct function of a person's state of fitness; the exercise which leaves an unfit person feeling stiff the following day may leave a fitter person unaffected. Sprains are less likely to occur following regular training, since the joints concerned become stronger and more capable of tolerating twists and shocks. Similarly, the body becomes more capable of resisting overuse injuries like stress fractures. Whilst it is true that overuse injuries occur in those who are highly trained, it takes considerable stress for this to happen. Regular training enables the body to tolerate much higher levels of exercise without the risk of overuse injury.

Besides these direct benefits on health, however, exercise has another major benefit. This is the way in which it contributes to weight control. Remember that keeping the right weight is a matter of obtaining the correct balance between the food you take in and the energy you use. In order to make sure that the balance is correct, it is necessary to pay attention to both diet and exercise. Only by exercising correctly and eating correctly can you be sure of keeping your weight how you want it.

Exercise is involved in weight control in two ways. The first, and most obvious way, is in directly burning up calories. To perform sustained exercise means placing extra demands on the body; these extra demands must be fuelled by burning up extra calories. Obviously, different kinds of exercises will burn up different amounts of calories, as will maintaining the exercise for different periods of time. Thus, running a mile will burn more calories than walking a mile; running 2 miles will burn more than running 1. By knowing a little about how different kinds of exercise use different amounts of fuel, it is possible to maintain a precise balance between the body's intake of fuel and the amount it uses. If your weight is not how you wish, it is possible to adjust the balance by changing either your food intake and/or your level of exercise as appropriate.

Regular exercise also has an effect on weight in addition to the direct burning off of calories whilst the exercise is being performed. Even when you are totally inactive your body still needs fuel to keep your normal bodily processes going – not only activities like breathing, circulation of the blood and so on, but also maintaining a certain state of readiness in the muscles. All of these require energy. The rate at which your body uses up energy in such processes is called the metabolic rate. A high metabolic rate uses up more energy, and therefore more calories, than a low metabolic rate. Metabolic rate varies at different times of the day, with different levels of activity and so on. Sleeping lowers metabolic rate, whilst eating produces a temporary rise. One of the effects of exercise is to produce a rise in metabolic rate not only during exercise but also during the remainder of the day. As a result, the person who exercises regularly is using up more calories even when resting than the person who does not.

Of course, this help in controlling weight, provided by exercise, is not merely a matter of looking better. Controlling your weight is an essential element of staying healthy. The woman who is the right weight is less likely to have problems with her heart, blood pressure problems, and problems like backache. She is more able to sustain effort and is thus less likely to become tired easily – and more able to perform the exercises necessary for good health.

### Particular benefits of exercise during pregnancy
Exercising correctly when you're pregnant means, of course, that you gain the same sort of benefits which we have just discussed. In addition, however, there are many ways in which exercise may be of especial benefit to the pregnant woman. Many women, for example, find that taking up regular exercise is a great help in giving up smoking. The general improvement in muscle tone which results from exercise can do much to prepare you for the difficulties of pregnancy and childbirth. In general, trained

athletes have been found to have much easier pregnancies than non-athletes, with fewer miscarriages and a shorter second stage of labour (during which the baby is pushed out through the birth canal). The value of exercise is now so widely recognised that instruction in exercise forms a routine part of ante-natal classes. It is worth looking more closely at some of the specific benefits which are possible.

*Strength*

As we mentioned earlier, exercise has amongst its effects the strengthening of the muscles involved. This extra strength does not necessarily mean noticeably bigger muscles; your strength can increase considerably before you notice that a muscle is larger. The extra strength of the muscles can, however, be of considerable value during pregnancy. Careful control of your weight in pregnancy will mean that you can expect to gain around 20 lb or so (9-10 kg) in total weight. Carrying this extra weight around will obviously be easier if the muscles involved are a little stronger. Remember that the extra weight you gain will be with you 24 hours a day; whilst it may not seem a great deal at first sight, without a little extra strength available to you, it will soon make its presence felt.

Besides its use in carrying around your extra weight, a little extra strength has other benefits. The extra weight doesn't only cause problems by being a little extra to carry around; it has to be carried in a particular way – mostly in front of your body. The effect of this is to move your centre of gravity forward in front of your pelvic girdle. This causes added difficulty for the muscles in your back, which need to 'pull back' in order to maintain balance. Without the strength to do this and still keep your back fairly straight, it can be tempting to simply pull back on your neck and shoulders, producing excessive curvature in the spine and contributing substantially to the risk of back problems.

The extra strength helps reduce the risk of back problems in another way as well. You'll remember that one of the effects of pregnancy is the softening of tendons and ligaments. Stretching of these fibres can be a major contribution to backache, by loosening the grip which the back muscles maintain on the joints of the spine. A stronger set of back muscles enables you to compensate for these effects, so that the risk of back problems is lessened. It is important to note that many back problems, once started, can be very persistent, and doctors treating these difficulties strongly believe that prevention is much better than cure.

Of course, back problems are sometimes caused by undue strain being placed on the muscles or joints involved; the changes in pregnancy may mean that you are much more susceptible to such strains. One of the ways in which these strains can be avoided is the use of correct lifting techniques. When picking something up from the floor it is important to do so by bending at the knees and keeping the back upright. Bending forward from the waist is extremely dangerous, and can place considerable strain on back muscles. The trouble is that many people find bending at the knees quite tiring. Once again, by strengthening the leg muscles involved, the correct lifting technique will become easier, making you much less likely to be tempted into using dangerous techniques like lifting from the waist.

Finally, it should be noted that the extra strength can also go a long way towards maintaining the shape you require. As we mentioned earlier, a muscle need not be large to be strong; a strong muscle will, however, be firm. This helps your shape in two ways. First, such firm muscle will keep its shape and won't wobble in the way that fat does. Second, the muscles will help to keep the rest of your body's tissues in the shape you want, giving support to your abdomen and other parts of your body. With strong muscles you can shape your body as you want it and hold it in that shape; you can't do the same with fat.

Clearly, then, the increased strength obtained through exercise can be of great value in pregnancy. It can help you carry the extra weight; it can help avoid problems like backache; and it can help you to maintain not only the weight but also the shape you desire.

*Stamina*
A further benefit of exercise is that besides making muscles stronger, it also increases their capacity for continued effort, that is to say, it improves their endurance (stamina). Like the increase in strength, this has a number of potential benefits to the pregnant woman, with perhaps the most obvious being the way in which

extra endurance enables you to cope with the additional weight you are carrying. Whilst pregnancy often produces a feeling of extra tiredness, particularly in the first trimester, this may be less of a problem for women who have developed good endurance by suitable exercise before conception. Even during pregnancy, however, it is still possible to develop endurance and obtain the resultant benefits. At the very least, you should be able to maintain the endurance or stamina you had before you were pregnant. You shouldn't 'go downhill' during the pregnancy. During the second trimester it is not uncommon for women to feel particularly well, and this can provide the opportunity to build up stamina and endurance in preparation for the time when weight is at its greatest and for childbirth itself – which everyone would agree puts tremendous demands on a woman's stamina.

The extra stamina is also of value when exercise is part of the overall programme of weight control. Whilst all forms of exercise will make some contributions to the overall balance between food intake and energy expenditure, it appears to be the case that the kind of exercise which is most useful in developing stamina is also the kind which contributes most to weight control. Jogging steadily or walking briskly for a fairly long distance, for example, is a good way of building up endurance – probably much better than running flat out for half a minute. Anyone who has noted the preponderance of slender figures running in the big city marathons like London will testify to the fact that relatively slow, long-distance jogging is also a very effective form of weight control – although fortunately, it's not necessary to run as far as marathon runners to gain the benefits.

Finally, of course, the extra stamina comes in useful in gaining the other benefits of exercise. If you have good endurance, not only will you be more able to cope with the exercises which are recommended, you will also find them easier and more enjoyable, and therefore be more likely to actually keep on doing them every time you should. Some exercise is going to be essential during pregnancy if you're going to come through it all with both yourself and your baby in good health. Developing your stamina makes it easier for you to do what you need in keeping the right balance of food and exercise.

*Suppleness*

Obviously suppleness is an advantage when giving birth, but as we have already explained, pregnancy itself produces an increase in suppleness. For most women there will be little, if any, need to do specific suppleness exercises, and for many, such exercises may carry particular risks unless done carefully and in conjunction with strengthening exercises. In Chapter 8 we discuss some of the ways in which exercises with a high premium on suppleness may safely be continued during pregnancy.

*Movement*

Surprising as it may seem, the very action of moving muscles during exercise has a number of benefits itself for the pregnant woman. The movement of muscles contributes to the pumping of blood around the body, reducing the amount of work the heart would otherwise have to do. This is one reason why exercises which do not involve actual movement of the muscle, like isometrics, may carry such risks as increased blood pressure. This assistance in blood circulation is particularly important during pregnancy when the changes in your body can leave you with increased risk of problems like varicose veins. Simply standing around in one place, for example by doing the washing up, means that the heart has to work hard to pump blood against the action of gravity from the feet back to the heart and lungs without any help from movement of the leg muscles. If, however, you spend the same amount of time walking or jogging, although the heart still has to pump the blood the same distance, the movement of the muscles in the legs helps with the pumping action, resulting in an easier blood flow. This results in reduced demand on the veins in the legs themselves and, in consequence, a reduced risk of varicose veins.

Just as the physical pumping action of the muscles provides a crude supplement to the pumping action of the heart, we can detect a similar benefit of movement in the digestive process. One of the most common problems of pregnancy can be chronic constipation, resulting from the relaxation of the smooth muscles inside the body which are normally responsible for pushing whatever we've eaten through the digestive system. When these muscles become less effective, the food is not pushed through the body as quickly and constipation results. Of course, this problem can be reduced by the adoption of a healthy diet with adequate fibre, and following the guidelines for eating given in this book will greatly reduce the tendency to constipation. In addition to the effect of a healthy diet, however, many women can reduce constipation by taking regular exercise. Just as the movement of the muscles provides a supplement to the pumping action of the heart, so the movement of the body provides a supplement to the pumping action of the muscles of the digestive system. The rhythmic movements of gentle jogging, or even walking briskly, for example, can do much to help the passage of whatever we've eaten so that it proceeds through the intestines normally, despite the reduced ability of the muscles of the digestive system. By adopting a sensible pattern of eating and doing sufficient exercise to supplement the smooth action within the body, it is possible to avoid the risk of constipation. What's more, solving the problem this way is both more healthy, and usually more effective, than consuming huge quantities of laxatives in the hope of temporary relief.

Finally, we should note that in addition to the benefits mentioned above, there are a number of other possible benefits to be gained from regular exercise. Exercises such as running and walking, for example, will usually take you out into the daylight. Even the minimum amount of sun your skin receives on an overcast winter's day can help in the production of some of the extra vitamin D supplies your body will need whilst pregnant. Indeed, since exercises (like running) may make you quite warm, you'll be able to go out into the sunlight wearing fewer clothes, meaning that more of your skin sees the sun, thus increasing the benefit – besides enabling you to start obtaining a tan when the sun is shining but the weather too cold for inactive sunbathing. Similarly, the fresh air you obtain is likely to make you feel better and healthier. On top of all this, most people find that after a period of exercise, it is much easier to relax. Since pregnancy is an exciting time, with a lot going on and people to visit, preparations to make and so on, it is often quite difficult simply to sit down and relax. Yet the ability to relax is of great importance. Exercise, for example, is of little use unless it is also combined with appropriate rest and relaxation to give the body time to reorganize in accordance with the extra demands that exercise makes. As we have mentioned, exercise itself can help with relaxation; in addition, there are a number of procedures especially designed to teach you to be able to relax. Before leaving the topic of exercise, therefore, it is worth paying a little attention to the other side of the coin – relaxation.

*Relaxation*
Whilst we often talk about relaxation, very few of us put a great deal of thought into what we actually mean by the term. For many people the term relaxation is used to describe whatever they do in their spare time; but if someone says that they, for example, play squash for relaxation, they clearly aren't talking about the same thing that most of us mean. For the present we can think of relaxation quite conveniently as simply the absence of tension. In fact, the term 'tension' here is surprisingly appropriate. By taking careful measurements with sensitive instruments, scientists have found that when we are tense we commonly have a slightly higher level of tension in many of our muscles. The increase in tension is often too slight to be noticeable in any single muscle, but when it affects several muscles, the result can be an overall feeling which we quite rightly describe as 'tension'.

One implication of this is that we can learn to relax if we can learn to eliminate the tension from the muscles – or at lest reduce it to a more reasonable level. Various ways of doing this have been developed, which commonly involve concentrating on one muscle at a time and relaxing the muscles one by one until an overall feeling of relaxation is obtained. Other approaches to relaxation training involve breathing exercises and a procedure called 'autogenic' training in which you learn to visualize and imagine particular scenes and circumstances in which you feel relaxed. By combining each of these procedures, it is possible to learn highly effective methods of relaxation. In addition, of course, many forms of exercise, particularly such procedures as yoga and dance, emphasize relaxation as part of their normal activities.

Relaxation is to be recommended for a number of reasons. At a general level, too much tension and too little relaxation has been associated with a number of medical problems, including heart disease, ulcers and similar problems. On the positive side, relaxation is, as we mentioned earlier, an essential element in obtaining the benefits of exercise, since it is during the relaxation that the body produces the changes in itself which permit it to cope with the added demands. Added to this, of course, is the fact that relaxation is a pleasant feeling, taking you away from your worries and producing a general feeling of well-being.

Relaxation also has a number of potential benefits with regard to common problems of pregnancy. Relaxation techniques have for example been found useful in treating some cases of insomnia, a problem which many women report, particularly in the third trimester. Relaxation can help in the lowering of blood pressure, which may be of particular importance if your blood pressure is higher than normal. The ability to relax can help you deal with any worries or concerns you may have during pregnancy; if you are unable to relax, such worries may make you so anxious that the anxiety interferes with your ability to deal with the problems. Finally, the ability to relax may be invaluable during labour, although it is unlikely that you will achieve total relaxation at such a time. Relaxation training is therefore an integral and important part of your plan for good health, and should be approached as thoroughly and systematically as the other parts.

## Summary

We have seen that pregnancy is for most women no reason to avoid exercise. Although there are some risks involved in exercise, it should not be forgotten that there are also risks in not exercising. For most women, exercise will be of considerable benefit if approached sensibly and carefully. Such benefits extend beyond the general benefits that exercise has for everyone, such as decreased risk of problems like coronary heart disease, to give help with several of the common problems of pregnancy. Thus, by exercising appropriately, a woman may reduce the chances of problems like backache, varicose veins, and constipation associated with pregnancy. In addition, she will feel more able to handle the demands of pregnancy, find it easier to maintain her shape and be more likely to finish her pregnancy with both her baby and herself in excellent health. Exercise may also supplement the specific training methods available to assist with relaxation, which is itself not only essential in enabling the body to benefit from the exercise, but also a possible aid to dealing with insomnia and, later, with the birth itself. By exercising and relaxing appropriately, it is possible, in conjunction with sensible eating patterns, to have a healthy baby and still maintain the shape you want.

# PART 2

# How to Control Your Weight During and After Pregnancy

# 6

# How to Achieve Self-Control

**Self-control: is it a skill that can be learned, or is it will-power?**

Now you have read Part 1 of this book, you should know quite a few things about being pregnant. We've given you a few tips on how to prepare for pregnancy (if you get the chance!). We've also described some of the major changes that happen to your body (Chapter 2), and what weight doctors recommend that you should aim to gain throughout the 40 weeks of pregnancy (Chapter 3). You've also been told some facts about nutrition (Chapter 4) and exercise (Chapter 5).

You should now therefore be fired with enthusiasm for starting a health programme which will be of maximum benefit for you and the developing baby. But where to begin? Perhaps you feel that following an eating regime slightly different from that which you're used to (maybe with less sugar, fat and salt than you normally eat) will tax your will-power too much. Or, it could be that you think you're basically a lazy type who doesn't much enjoy exercise and really couldn't be bothered with trying to keep the muscles in trim whilst pregnant. But remember, you have a responsibility not only to yourself now, but also to the baby inside you. This baby is totally dependent on you. Therefore, it's absolutely essential, if you want to do the best thing for your child, that you keep yourself healthy. The correct mixture of a good, well-balanced eating plan, appropriate exercise, and relaxation, is the best way of ensuring that you stay as fit as possible. If you want to maximize the chances of having a healthy baby, you have to be a healthy mother.

So, let us say that you've made up your mind to make every effort to become fit and healthy. It doesn't matter one bit if you think you are 'weak-willed'. Will-power is an odd thing: please don't think of it as something that you're either born with, or you're not. Anybody can acquire the skill to tackle a task and to accomplish it. You can learn the best way to achieve your goals. If you like to think of this in terms of will-power, then you can learn how to develop will-power by learning to tackle your problems in a special way, that will ensure that you accomplish the tasks you set yourself.

For example, let us say your task is to give up eating so many sweet things. If you decide that as from now, or tomorrow, you will *never* touch sugary foods again, then you will almost certainly fail to achieve this goal. The problem is NOT that you don't have strong enough will-power. The problem is, simply, that you are asking too much of yourself. You are setting yourself an unrealistic goal. A task is much easier to tackle if you break it down into manageable pieces (or mini-goals) and then deal with each mini-goal separately. Try to enjoy the process; feel you've accomplished something each time you overcome a part of the problem. For instance, if you want to give up sugary things, how should you do this? First of all, write down how often you normally eat these things. You might find that you like biscuits, say four times a day with a cup of tea. Your first mini-goal might be to have only one biscuit with each of the four cups of tea (therefore you have only four biscuits in total in the day). Your next mini-goal might be to have only three biscuits a day. When a few days have passed, and you feel comfortable with three biscuits a day, you might go on to have only two biscuits a day, then after a while, have a sweet treat just once a day. Replace the biscuits with other, more nutritious, foods, so you don't feel deprived. But, perhaps your life would be miserable without biscuits at least three times a day? Perhaps you just don't want to do without them at all? Rather than try to forego them entirely, why not bake your own, with dried fruit, nuts, wholemeal flour, and just a little fat? With plenty of dried fruit, there should be no need to add sugar. If you can't cut something out of your diet, why not try to replace it with a low sugar (or non-sugar) healthier variety of the same thing?

So, if you think you have little or no will-power, it doesn't matter at all. The trick is to learn how to approach your problems in such a way that you achieve success. We are going to describe a few general principles which will help you tackle your problems, help you make the changes in your life style that you want, and achieve self-control.

## Principles of self-control

*Break a problem down into manageable pieces*
It could well be that all the advice we have given about diet, exercise and relaxation, will mean you need to make some big changes. We have just given you a simple, single example, of a woman trying to cut down the sugar she eats by reducing her biscuit consumption. However, we've asked you, earlier in the book, to cut down on sugar *and* fat *and* salt. We've also asked you to increase the fibre in your diet. In addition, your exercise and relaxation habits need to be reconsidered. These are a great many changes to make all at once. You might decide to make a *slow* start in tackling all of these areas, and that is fine. But if you decide that, as from now, you are a changed person, with a totally different life style, you'll probably fail. The temptation is to be so full of good intentions that you ask too much of yourself. You vow never to touch sugar again. You throw out the salt cellar, the butter, the lard, the bag of sugar, and the jars of jam. You buy an extra large bag of bran for fibre. You say you'll exercise much more, planning to go for a run or a swim every day. If you're lucky you'll stick with these good intentions for a week or maybe even a month. Nearly everyone lapses very quickly though. And once you give up on one thing, the temptation is to give up on all of them.

It is much better to approach your ultimate goal gradually and make lots of small, easy changes over a period of weeks. For example, to begin with, you might find you want to cut out sugar from just some meals or snacks. Or you might like to bake low sugar (or non-sugar) biscuits or cakes of your own. There again, you might decide to keep your consumption of sweet foods the same for now, but first tackle your consumption of sweet drinks, cutting down on sweet fizzy drinks and sugar in tea and coffee. Your next aim might be to go further than cutting sweet drinks down, and actually cut them right out. Only then might you go on to reduce sugar in food. Do what YOU find easiest first. Then go for the next easiest thing, and so on.

*At the same time* you are reducing sugar consumption, do what you find easiest to reduce fat and salt. Now, if you are cutting down sugar by eating less cake, biscuits or chocolate, you will automatically be eating less fat! However, if you are cutting down on sugar by not adding it to any of your drinks, then tackle your fat problem directly. You might like to try a low fat spread, such as 'Gold' or 'Outline'. Or spread your usual choice of butter or margarine a little more thinly on bread. Alternatively, you might simply start to reduce your fat consumption by frying food a little less often, or having white fish or chicken (both are low in fat) a little more often instead of red meat. Start with the thing you find easiest to do. When that's conquered, go on to the next thing.

Of course, as well as reducing fat and sugar, you will, at the same time, be wanting to reduce salt. Perhaps you might start slowly, and week by week gradually reduce the amount you use in cooking. Alternatively, start with reducing the salt you add at table. Perhaps you might fill the salt cellar with a mixture of your usual salt plus a potassium salt, such as 'Ruthmol'. Then you can phase out the amount of ordinary salt in the salt cellar until eventually it contains only the potassium salt. Again, do what you find easiest first.

Similarly, you must work out the easiest ways for you, personally, to include more fibre in your diet. Try to build an exercise and also a relaxation programme into your daily regime. Don't be *over* ambitious with any of the changes you plan to make. So, to begin with, set yourself a mini-goal for each of the six tasks you have set yourself, reducing sugar, reducing fat, reducing salt, increasing fibre, increasing exercise, learning to relax. Each of these six tasks needs to be broken down into realistic steps (mini-goals) that you feel pretty sure you can accomplish with very little effort. Although we will be showing you, later in the book, how to best work out your mini-goals, here is a small example of how to set out a list of mini-goals for reducing sugar intake.

*An example: how to reduce sugar intake*

The woman in this example would usually have quite a bit of sugar in her normal diet. A typical pattern of eating for her would be:

6 cups of tea during the day, with *2 spoons* of sugar in *each* cup

breakfast: *2 spoons* of sugar on breakfast cereal and milk
*1 spoon* of marmalade on toast, with butter too.

mid-morning: *2 biscuits*

lunch: usually savoury sandwiches (Monday to Friday) a savoury snack on Saturday, and a roast meal on Sunday
sometimes lunch includes a *cake*, or some *biscuits*, or a *sweet dessert* of some kind (4 or 5 days of the week)

mid-afternoon: a *sweet snack*

dinner: a savoury meal
sometimes a *sweet dessert*

evening: perhaps a few *sweets* or *chocolate* whilst watching television.

This isn't a full example of this woman's diet. We haven't written in all the specific foods, and the exact portions. However, there is enough in this little example to see that this woman is eating sugar very often during the day. We have emphasized the *obvious* times sugar is taken, either added to foods or drinks, or already present in foods.

Rather than try to cut out sugar entirely, all in one go, a realistic series of mini-goals for this woman would be:

| week | mini-goal | *ways to reduce sugar* |
|---|---|---|
| 1 | 1 | only 1 spoon of sugar in drinks |
| 2 | 2 | sweet dessert of any kind, with lunch, only 2 days a week |
| 3 | 3 | just 1 biscuit mid-morning |
| 4 | 4 | bake some sugar-free biscuits, and have 1 mid-morning and 1 mid-afternoon |
| 5 | 5 | only ½ spoon sugar in drinks |
| 6 | 6 | sweet dessert with dinner, only 2 days a week |
| 7 | 7 | no sugar in drinks |
| 8 | 8 | no sweets or chocolate whilst watching television; if hungry before going to bed, have a small, savoury snack |
| 9 | 9 | only 1 spoon of sugar on breakfast cereal. |

You can see that this person is having much less sugar by the end of week 9 when all the mini-goals have been achieved. She is still having some sugar, but she feels she is the kind of person that likes sweet things so much that she doesn't want to give up sugar and sugary foods entirely. And there is really no reason why she shouldn't have the occasional treat. But you can clearly see that by the time *all* the mini-goals have been achieved, the main goal (a large reduction of sugar intake) has been reached.

Of course, this is just an example. You have to discover for yourself your own particular eating pattern and then work out a list of your own mini-goals. Start with the easiest thing first and make this mini-goal 1. The next easiest thing will be mini-goal 2, and so on. Do remember that when you achieve mini-goal 1 and go on to mini-goal 2, you still have to include mini-goal 1 as well as number 2. When you go to mini-goal 3, you should still be including mini-goals 1 and 2, and so on, so that by the end of the list you are completing all the mini-goals all of the time.

The woman in our example took 1 week with each mini-goal but you may take longer if you wish. You do not need to spend the same amount of time with each mini-goal. Move on when you feel comfortable with your level and feel that it's time to progress. If you find that you get stuck on one of the mini-goals, try to break it down into easier pieces. For example, your mini-goal might be to have 1 spoon of sugar in your tea instead of 2. If you find that this tastes just horrible, then set yourself a less difficult mini-goal of 1½ spoons of sugar in your tea. When you've accomplished this for a week or so, move on to the next obvious step of just 1 spoon of sugar in each drink.

You will need to set yourself a list of mini-goals for each of the tasks we have set you, reducing sugar, salt and fat, and increasing fibre; doing more exercise, and learning to relax. We will show you in more detail how to set mini-goals for more than one task, in the next chapter.

### Set realistic goals

Many people set themselves unrealistic goals. What are your ultimate aims? You want to have a healthy pregnancy. You may want to adopt some good eating habits, and do more exercise of the right type. Fine. You can do these things and still indulge in the odd treat. If someone gives you a box of chocolates, there is no need to give them away, or to binge them all in one day to 'get rid of the temptation'. Try to incorporate them into your eating regime at times that you allow yourself a little treat (perhaps have a couple of chocolates after dinner occasionally). If you love sugary, fatty and salty foods, don't make yourself miserable by trying to do without them entirely, then having a binge on forbidden foods and feeling guilty. All we want you to do is to retrain your appetite slightly, and permanently, so that you are genuinely not quite as fond, nor as dependent, on fatty, sugary and salty foods, as you were.

With exercise it is also important to set realistic goals, especially during pregnancy. It is highly desirable for you to keep your abdominal muscles in good shape, and to retain good posture. Keep generally active (providing there are no medical complications) throughout pregnancy. Go for walks, go swimming, or whatever takes your fancy and that is safe (see Chapter 8 for advice on this). However, this is not the time to start training to run a marathon, or over-exerting yourself. There is no point in being unrealistic. Don't make out a list of mini-goals which demand that you swim 20 lengths of the pool each day in week 1; 30 lengths of the pool each day in week 2; 40 lengths of the pool each day in week 3, and so on. Set mini-goals which you are likely to achieve and that you will enjoy. It is better to make a thing too easy than too hard. For example, if you are not a very active person, your mini-goal for week 1 might simply be to go for a 10-minute walk each day. Then, if you find that on one day in week 1 you really feel like a longer walk of, say, 30 minutes, then have a longer walk! Enjoy yourself, but don't over-do things. Don't, however, think that by walking 30 minutes on one day, you needn't have your 10-minute walk on the next 2 days. If your aim is to get out for a 10-minute walk each day of the week, then you should go, for at least 10 minutes, on *each* day. If you really feel that you cannot make a walk each day, then do not set the mini-goal for each day. You can, of course, specify exactly how many days in the week you wish to exercise. The point is, that whatever you have set, you should try to stick to it. The only exception to this rule is if you find you are feeling unwell or experiencing the extreme tiredness often associated with the first and last stages of pregnancy. Let yourself off exercise if you honestly think you are unwell or overtired (but remember to start again when the symptoms pass!)

*Make it easy to review your progress*
What we are saying is that you should make changes very gradually in order to achieve success. The problem is that you may well lose track of your progress unless you write things down. We are asking you to change lots of things, the sugar, fat, salt and fibre that you eat, and also the amount of exercise and relaxation periods you have. It's no use jotting down lists of mini-goals in the margin of a magazine, or on the back of your shopping list, because the chances are that you will lose them. So, buy yourself a diary with a fairly large space for writing in each day. If it's not the time of year when diaries are in the shops, buy a large writing book and write out your own daily headings. We are not suggesting you spend all your time writing down everything you eat or drink. But a diary is useful in many ways. At the beginning of your diary write down your list of mini-goals for each thing you want to change – sugar, fat, salt, fibre, exercise and relaxation. There needn't be the same number of mini-goals for each thing; use more mini-goals for the harder things. Once you've written all your lists at the beginning of the diary (and we'll be giving you more details of how to do this in the next chapter), it's time to start on changing your habits. Take the first, easiest mini-goal for each of the tasks and write them down in the space for Monday of the first week you are starting your health campaign. Here is an example:

*week 1  Monday  mini-goals for this week*

| | |
|---|---|
| mini-goal 1 for sugar: | only 1 spoon of sugar in drinks |
| mini-goal 1 for fat: | try a low-fat margarine, like 'Gold' or 'Outline' |
| mini-goal 1 for salt: | use only ½ the usual amount in cooking |
| mini-goal 1 for fibre: | try wholemeal bread for 3 days of the week |
| mini-goal 1 for exercise: | go for a 10-minute walk each day |
| mini-goal 1 for relaxation: | relax on bed for 10 minutes each day |

Then, for the rest of the week you could simply record whether you are keeping to your mini-goals. If you don't much like writing, just put a tick in the slot in the diary for that particular day, if that day was a success and you kept to all your mini-goals. But try to write down if you are having any particular difficulties, or even if you are finding it too easy! Perhaps you find you are really tired one day and so you missed going for a walk. This is perfectly permissible. Try to be aware of what your body is trying to 'tell' you to do. Write down anything that you feel is important to you. At the end of the week you can review how you've done. Did you succeed with everything, everyday? If you did, then you can move on to mini-goal 2 for each task in week 2. However, if there was a mini-goal that you were not always successful with, then stay with this mini-goal for another week. For example, if you only went for a 10-minute walk on 3 days, stay with mini-goal 1 during week 2, and try to keep to it this time; of course, if you were successful with all the other mini-goals in week 1, then you could continue with mini-goal 2 for all these others in week 2. So your mini-goals for week 2 might look like this:

*week 2   Monday   mini-goals for this week*

| | |
|---|---|
| mini-goal 2 for sugar: | have sweet dessert with lunch on only 2 days |
| mini-goal 2 for fat: | fried food on 2 days in the week |
| mini-goal 2 for salt: | use only a tiny shake of salt at table |
| mini-goal 1 for exercise: | go for a 10-minute walk each day |
| mini-goal 2 for relaxation: | have a relaxing bath, with a favourite bath-oil each evening before bed |

Don't forget that when you move on to another mini-goal you still do all the things specified in the previous mini-goals. So, in this example, as well as doing the things you've listed for the week, you also do all the things you did the week before.

You should continue making progress as we have showed you. At the beginning of each week, write down your new mini-goal for each task. When you've come to the end of your list of mini-goals for a particular task (say, reducing sugar intake), then you've obviously accomplished a great deal. Your aim will then be to hold at this level for this task. It shouldn't be too long before you get through the list of mini-goals for each thing you are working at.

You will have succeeded in cutting down sugar, fat and salt, and increasing fibre; you also should be happy with your progress with exercise and relaxation. Once you've worked through all your mini-goals and thus achieved your ultimate goal with all these things it is then important to maintain your progress. You don't want to backslide!

A diary is also useful for recording a number of other things, such as your weight, and your 'vital statistics' (which should prove very interesting whilst you are pregnant!) So it is worth continuing with the diary at least until the baby is born. It should be an interesting and happy reminder of your pregnancy.

*Reward yourself for success*
Every little mini-goal that you reach should be regarded as a great success and worth a reward. Just reading your weekly progress in your diary can actually be a very good reward. But there is no reason why you shouldn't add to this if you wish. Give yourself a little treat at the end of each successful week. Perhaps you'd appreciate a trip to the cinema? Or, you could buy yourself something you'd like, perhaps some fancy bath-oil, or some interesting magazines to read, as part of your relaxation period. If money is a bit short and you feel guilty about spending it on yourself, then you could always buy a little toy or a small article of clothing for the baby you are carrying! Alternatively, (or even, as well as this) you could make a chart and reward yourself with points (one point for each mini-goal achieved). When you've got a certain number of points you can give yourself a very big treat (or better still, get your husband or a friend to co-operate and give you that big treat when you've earned enough points).

*Do not punish yourself for failure*
If you achieve only some, or even none, of your mini-goals one week, do not feel you have failed. Expect setbacks occasionally. Try to analyse just why you failed. Were you asking yourself to make too much progress this week? Was the pregnancy making you feel extra tired or extra sick? Was it a holiday period when you found it less easy to maintain control? Any of these things can happen. If disaster strikes one week, do *not* try to be super good the next week to make up for it. Don't place even more demands on yourself. Instead, look back in your diary to the last mini-goal

you did achieve for each thing. Try these mini-goals again. When you are successful with them for another week, then progress to a slightly higher level by going for the next mini-goal for each item. Never ask too much of yourself. It could be that with some mini-goals you need to spend much longer than a week with them before you feel comfortable enough to progress further. Feel free to do this.

It could be that you really get stuck with a mini-goal and simply can't progress further. If this is the case, it suggests that the jump to the next mini-goal is just too big for you. You will then have to review your list of mini-goals and put in some even easier mini-goals that you *can* achieve.

*Make things as easy and enjoyable for yourself as you can*
It should be fun to work your way through the mini-goals you have set yourself. They should make the changes in your habit patterns easy to make, and you should therefore feel a real sense of achievement with each week that passes.

Don't forget to look back at some of the tips we gave you towards the end of Chapter 4. Remember to *plan* your nutritious meals and snacks, and try not to eat between these planned events. Focus on enjoying the food you eat during your meals and snacks; don't just grab or nibble at food whilst doing something else, like watching television. Never eat unless you are hungry. Don't feel guilty about leaving food.

All these general principles of self-control should help you to control your weight. Don't forget that you should be careful to record your weight in your diary, every day if possible. If you are in the first 13 or 14 weeks of pregnancy, you should aim to stay roughly the same weight. Thereafter, you should gain about 1 lb (0.45 kg) a week until about week 37. Write your weekly weight aim at the beginning of each week, along with your mini-goals for that week.

Concentrating on a good, well-balanced food regime, and doing exercise, should, in itself, help considerably with your weight control. The basic principle of weight control is that total energy derived from your food intake should equal your own energy needs (energy to keep you generally 'ticking over' plus energy for daily activities, including the energy needed to support

the baby when you are pregnant). Any extra fuel, taken in addition
to this, will be turned into fat. (If you don't take in enough fuel,
you will start to use your fat stores to supply you with energy.) So,
if you find you're putting on too much weight, it means that
your food intake is supplying you with more fuel than is needed
for your energy needs and the energy needs directly associated
with the pregnancy. The surplus fuel is therefore turned into fat.
You should therefore try to eat a little less, or exercise a little more
(to use up the extra fuel), or perhaps a bit of both. Your weight will
tell you whether you are balancing things properly.

## Tools of self-control

We have already mentioned some tools of self-control when we
were talking about general principles. There are probably a great
many things that you might use to help you, but we are going to
mention some of the most useful ones.

### Diary

One of the most important tools is your diary. It is absolutely
essential for you to record your progress. You need to know you
can keep track of where you are with your mini-goals for each thing
you are trying to change. A diary is useful to remind you of your
successes. And, if you are having difficulties, you should be able to
analyse just where you are going wrong, and then be able to put it
right, as we explained in the last section. You can write down figures,
such as your weight and body measurements. The diary is an aid to
change; it should enable you to get to know yourself better.

We have said that we believe the way to permanent success in
changing your habits for the better, is to make the process *easy* and
*fun*. This may sound like common sense. Yet how many people try
this method? Think of all those people who, every January 1st, set
themselves New Year's Resolutions (sometimes the same ones
year after year). These resolutions usually last just a few weeks at
most. People tend to set themselves very difficult goals. They
don't use a system of mini-goals. Most often they fail to achieve
their big goals. Or, if they *do* achieve them, the process is arduous
and gruelling, and then they very often backslide and end up at
square one again.

The principles we have described will help you towards a

permanent change in eating and exercise patterns generally. And what better time to start to obtain healthy habits like these than during your pregnancy? Now, some people may think our method is just too slow. Indeed, you are making such tiny changes that you may not really notice at first that you are getting anywhere at all. That is why it is so important to have a diary where all the tiny changes are listed down. You can look through it and reassure yourself that, provided you make all the tiny, easy changes you have planned, you will eventually achieve all of your major goals. A diary is a reminder of where you are heading! Finally, don't forget that your diary should be a lovely memento of a happy, healthy pregnancy

*Weighing machine*
*Do* invest in a really good weighing machine. If you are getting weighed, say, every month at the ante-natal clinic, this is not enough to help you adjust your food intake on a regular enough basis to keep to your target weight aim. So, you must get some weighing scales. Go to a shop where they have several well-known brand names, and try them out if possible. Step on and off the scales two or three times, and make sure they register the same weight every time! You want a good, reliable weighing machine. *Which?* magazine occasionally reviews weighing machines; you might like to find which ones they favour. (If you don't take this magazine, your local library should keep copies or be able to order ones for you.)

Perhaps you might like to invest in the newest type of scales, which give you your weight in numbers (a digital display), rather than leaving you to decide which particular place the pointer is at on the scale. If you don't have the money to buy weighing scales, either borrow some or locate your nearest public machine. Weigh every day if you possibly can, preferably at the same time of the day, and wearing the same amount of clothing.

Many experts recommend that you weigh once a week, but we are asking you to weigh each day. Why is this? It is a fact that your weight does fluctuate quite a bit during the day. Obviously, you will weigh more dressed than undressed. You will weigh more after you've eaten or drunk something. You will weigh less after a trip to the lavatory, or if you've been doing exercise or it is hot, and you have been sweating a lot. These changes in weight will not reflect a loss in fat or a gain in fat. The reason we ask you to weigh under the same conditions each day (for example, when you get up in the morning, before you eat or drink anything, and after you have been to the lavatory) is to try and get an accurate assessment of how you and the baby are really progressing. But even if you weigh under the same conditions each day, you might still get a relatively sudden change of about 3 lb (1.35 kg) from one day to the next. If you've had a salty meal, you might find you suddenly seem to gain a lot of weight overnight. Of course, this is just because the salt makes you retain water. When not pregnant, you may retain extra fluid just before your period is due. If you are constipated you will weigh more. Because of all these factors, some people think that the most realistic guide is to weigh once a week. However, we want you to weigh each day in order that you try to better understand your weight changes. If you gain 3 lb (1.35 kg) overnight, ask yourself why. Did you overeat slightly? Are you constipated? Did you eat an unusually salty meal which is making you retain water? Try to pinpoint a possible reason for the change. One happy thought you might like to bear in mind is that it is virtually IMPOSSIBLE to put on 3 lb (1.35 kg) of *fat* in one day. Why? To put on 1 lb (0.45 kg) of fat you need to eat 3,500 calories. Therefore, to gain three times this amount of fat you'd need to eat a surplus of 3 x 3,500 = 10,500 calories worth of food. These calories would need to be taken *as well as* what you'd normally eat to supply you with your energy for the day. So, if you normally need 2,000 calories a day, you need to eat a total of 12,500 calories in the day in order to suddenly put on 3 lb (1.35 kg) of fat. If you look through a calorie booklet you'll appreciate that it would be almost impossible for someone to eat this much. 12,500 calories is roughly equivalent to *forty* 'Mars' bars! So, don't be overly disturbed by a sudden increase in weight. If you think it's caused by a salty meal, be extra careful with salt intake the next day. If you ate too many sugary things, cut back to normal. If you think you gained weight because you ate too much generally, try to revert to your usual amount. Don't decide you'll make up for any extra by eating hardly anything the day after a sudden weight gain. You'll find that by late afternoon you'll become ravenous, and you'll do the most human thing and eat everything in sight! We don't want you to overtax yourself and then lose control.

You'll probably find a big, sudden increase in weight, will go again just as suddenly as it came. Try to be objective in trying to understand your own particular weight change from day to day.

### Tape measure

Your bust, waist and hip measurements will obviously change. If, from the time you discover you are pregnant, you measure yourself every 2 or 3 weeks, you'll be able to see just which bits of you alter, and when. Your bust should start to get bigger first. As we described in Chapter 2, the womb is so small that it can't even be felt growing up into the abdomen until week 12. So, your waist measurements should not really increase by much, if at all, in the first trimester. If you find that your waist becomes much bigger early in pregnancy, you may be putting on unnecessary fat (in which case your weight will increase too). So beware, and take corrective action; if you are overeating, reduce to your normal amount. However, a more likely explanation for a sudden, large increase in waist measurement early in pregnancy is that you are constipated. So try to remedy this by increasing your fibre and liquid consumption.

The tape measure can be a very useful indicator of whether you are gaining body fat. As well as measuring bust, waist and hips, also measure around the top of your arm, around the top of your thigh, just above your knee, your calf and your ankle. Try to measure at the same point each time. If you find your arm and all your leg measurements becoming much bigger, then be wary! You're probably eating far too much. Look back at the chapter on food and pregnancy to remind yourself how much you should be eating. If your arm and leg measurements stay about the same size, but your ankles become bigger, this indicates excess water retention. Are you still eating too much salt? Are you remembering to sit with your feet up? Can you do more to avoid standing still?

Record your measurements in your diary. They are yet another way for you to monitor your progress. They give you information which will help you adjust your eating, exercise and relaxation habits appropriately.

### Charts

If you wish, you can keep charts or graphs of your progress. For example, you might keep a graph of your weight. Mark on the graph in pencil what your weight should be (your aim). then use a coloured pen to mark on the actual weight. Use a graph to cover you for the whole 40 weeks of pregnancy, and mark on your weekly weight aim. Look back to Chapter 3 to remind yourself how much you should aim to put on, and when. If you are not spot on target, do not worry overly about it. But if you are more than 2-3 lb (about 1-1½ kg) off course, you should take corrective action to make sure this trend does not continue. Make slight adjustments to your food intake and exercise to make sure that you don't go *too* far from your target. Never take drastic action, like starving yourself if you go a little above your aim, or eating non-stop if you go a little under. If you end the 40 weeks of pregnancy within about 7 lb (3.2 kg) of your target you will have done very well!

We mentioned earlier in this chapter that you might like to award yourself points for each mini-goal attained. You could chart or graph the number of points you collect. Or, perhaps you'd like to make a chart out to record your body measurements. This sort of thing may appeal very much to some of you. But if you are the type that doesn't like too much fuss with charts, graphs, and paper and pencil work generally, don't feel obliged to make out charts and graphs. Just use your diary.

*Camera*

If you own a camera, you might find it interesting to have photographs taken of yourself throughout the pregnancy. Have them taken every two or three weeks during the second and third trimesters. Perhaps you could have a photography session after you've been measuring yourself with the tape measure? Have one photo taken with you facing the camera, and one of you standing sideways. Wear as little in the photographs as you feel comfortable in, but remember that the object is to show your changing shape, so wearing an enormous tent-dress is not going to help you do this! These photographs should not only be a memento of the pregnancy, they should also be helping you to get a realistic view of yourself, aiding you in your resolve to have a healthy pregnancy and not put on more than the medically recommended amount of weight. What the photographs *should* show is that your bust is bigger and that your abdomen increases in size. What they *should not* show is that you are degenerating into an enormous, puffy balloon, with a double chin, fat arms, and fat and swollen legs. It is very easy to turn a blind eye to the fact that you are getting too fat if you are hidden away in maternity clothes. If you take regular photographs which show clearly how you are changing, you cannot easily ignore it if they show you are becoming too fat, and you can take appropriate action to prevent the situation getting wildly out of control.

If you can't afford to have photographs taken regularly (or if the idea just doesn't appeal to you) then make sure you have an honest look at yourself at regular intervals (preferably in a full length mirror) and try to decide whether you are looking fit and healthy and pregnant, or whether there are any problems.

## Methods of self-control
We have already mentioned, in passing, the methods of self-control we want you to use. Here is a summary of them.

### Self-monitoring
You should be aware of how the pregnancy is affecting your body. Your eating habits, and the amount of exercise and relaxation you have, will all combine to help make your pregnancy either healthy or unhealthy. It is essential for you to keep track of your own patterns of eating, relaxation and exercise. That is why we have stressed that you use a diary for monitoring progress. It will contain your lists of mini-goals; you'll be able to see just how things are going. You can assess how your body is changing shape by recording measurements. You are 'keeping an eye' on yourself. There is no more important time to do this than during pregnancy.

### Goal-setting
We have already explained how to break a big goal down into lots of mini-goals. A vague promise to try to do all the right things is not good enough. Specific targets have to be set for each individual week. Remember, you should always aim for what you think you can achieve. Don't set impossible tasks. Better to find that what you've set yourself is too easy, and that you can manage to do a little more than the mini-goal requires, rather than find that you can't achieve your mini-goal.

*Scheduling and forward planning*

Although in any one week you should only be concerned with your mini-goals, and your weight for that week, don't forget that this is a small step in a much larger plan. In any single week not a great deal should happen. You won't look really much different at week 16 than you did at week 15. And you won't look much different at week 36 than you did at week 35. Yet, all the tiny changes mount up over the weeks. You should certainly look very different at week 36 than you did at week 16! The small things you do every day, in trying to keep to your weekly mini-goals, really will mount up. The tiny improvements in eating, exercise and relaxation habits will add up to big improvements by the time the baby is born. But, you will need to remind yourself at times that these small weekly improvements really are worth making. You will need to look again at your lists of mini-goals at the beginning of your diary. We have deliberately asked you to plan ahead, scheduling all the mini-goals you want to achieve week by week, so that you *can* look ahead, beyond the small changes you are making at any one time. Think what an overall, enormous change for the better it will be when you've achieved *all* of your mini-goals.

*Keeping in tune with bodily needs*

It is, unfortunately, true that many of us stop using our own internal signals which are there to guide us into healthy ways of behaving. We don't always eat when we're hungry. We eat because it's a meal time, or perhaps we've been tempted by something delicious, or because we're bored, or because food comforts us. If we *do* start eating because we're hungry, we often don't stop when the hunger goes. We stop when the food is finished. We also may not always eat the food our body needs. We should think more about whether we really want fish, or cheese, or something else, in order to satisfy our hunger most at any particular eating time. It is very difficult to appreciate any strong hunger for a particular food if the appetite is being constantly dampened by a succession of sweet snacks, such as an endless stream of sugary drinks and biscuits throughout the day.

Although we suggest you plan the number of occasions each day that you want to sit and eat (you might plan three meals plus two nutritious snacks for example), we do *not* mean that you should be completely rigid in following set menus. Instead, you can adapt the food you eat to satisfy your particular fancy at the time. For example, you may have planned a fish meal for one evening, and a chicken meal for the next. However, if you really want chicken on the first night, although you planned to have fish, then have it. If you'd planned to follow the meal with an orange, but then having eaten it, you are really genuinely hungry for another one, then have it. If you planned to have salmon sandwiches on a particular lunchtime, but then you find the bread has gone stale (or someone has already eaten the salmon!), you will just have to improvise and eat something else. Choose any alternative food which is in line with the kind of healthy eating ideas we discussed in Chapter 4.

People do not normally write out a detailed menu for the whole week. However, they might think of the kinds of meals they could be eating. Most people do the bulk of their shopping just once a week, so they automatically plan ahead to some extent, because they buy food to make meals for a number of days. This is really all we want *you* to do. But plan to stock up with the types of food we have recommended rather than fatty and sugary foods. Buy *more* fish, chicken, rice, spaghetti, and pulses (peas and beans); buy less red meat. Try a low fat spread rather than butter. Try some sunflower oil rather than lard. Forget to pick up cakes and buy some wholemeal flour, nuts and dried fruit instead. Have a wholegrain cereal for breakfast rather than one which is sugar coated. Have lots of fruit and vegetables. It may seem strange at first to be loading your shopping trolley with some different foods. People tend to buy more or less the same things week after week. As we said earlier, you'll probably need to make these changes gradually. But *do* put some thought into what you bring back from your weekly trip to the shops; it will obviously be a major determining factor in what you eat during the week. And a final tip is never to do your shopping when you are extremely hungry. You are likely to find yourself loading your shopping trolley with all sorts of things which you really shouldn't have!

Please note, though, that although you might swop menus a little, don't eat outside of the occasions you'd planned to eat. If you plan to have three main meals, plus a nutritious snack mid-afternoon and before you go to bed, then don't eat between these times unless you are suffering from pregnancy sickness, in which case, nibble dry toast or crispbread whenever you feel the need. You can, however, have a drink whenever you wish (without sugar if possible). You should have plenty of fluid whilst you are pregnant. But try really hard to prevent yourself from absent-mindedly nibbling at food, for example, whilst preparing a meal, or when watching television. If you find you are always getting very hungry between your meals, either eat slightly larger meals or plan an extra, nutritious snack or two as part of your everyday eating routine. However, instead of finding you haven't planned enough eating occasions in the day, it is possible that you have planned too many. Never eat if you're not hungry. If you don't really want a meal or a snack that you had planned, then delay it slightly until you *are* hungry. If you planned a snack around, say, 4 o'clock in the afternoon and you find you just don't get hungry until about 6 o'clock, shortly before you'd planned to eat your evening meal, then miss the snack out altogether. It's perfectly permissible to omit a meal or snack if you're genuinely not hungry. The only time you should be careful to make yourself eat is if you find your hunger seems to disappear *entirely* and you start to fall below your weekly target weight. Even so, the loss of a *little* weight early in pregnancy isn't unusual and is nothing to worry about. However, try to maintain a slow and steady weight gain (around 1 lb or 0.45 kg a week) from the end of week 14 to about week 37.

You should also try to be aware of internal signals about your need for exercise and relaxation. If you'd planned a walk, or any activity, but find you are genuinely exhausted, then don't go. Have a relaxation period instead. You might always feel like a walk later on. However, if you'd planned a walk and it's just started to rain, don't use tiredness as an excuse. Go, and take an umbrella!

### Calorie counting spotchecks
We are not asking you to count up the calories in every food you eat. However, if you find that you are gaining too much weight, it can be useful to take a typical day's food and drink and work out how many calories you are consuming. It could well be that you

will be amazed. Most women should not be going above 2,400-2,500 calories or so a day in the second and third trimesters. So, if your score is a long way above this you'll have a very clear explanation for your weight gain. Calorie counting spotchecks can be useful, if done just occasionally, as added information which might help you adjust your eating habits appropriately.

However, if you don't like calorie counting, or if you know nothing about it, then there is no need to bother with this. If your weight is going up too much, eat less (and/or exercise more). If you are not gaining enough, eat more. Because you are weighing each day, you are never going to receive a really nasty shock at how different your weight is from what you thought it was. You'll see if you are going slightly away from target and therefore be able to make the slight alterations in eating and exercise habits necessary to keep weight under control.

# 7

# Getting The Food Right

Before you can begin to 'get the food right' you have to feel confident that you have the self-control necessary to do this. The last chapter explained just how easy it is to achieve your goals provided you use the right methods and the right tools. It is essential that you have read the last chapter *really thoroughly* before you begin to try to change your eating patterns in order to control your weight.

**Weight control: the first steps**
By now you should have read Chapter 4 and so have learned about foods to eat for maximum health. And, having read Chapter 6, you should also know *how* to set about changing your eating habits. However, the first steps in habit change are very important and it is essential that you tackle them in the right way.

It's probable that you haven't yet bought your diary (or note book). So, when are you going to do it? Tomorrow? The weekend? Try to buy your diary within *1 week* of reading this. What are you going to do until you have your diary and you can really get started? People tend to do one of two things, both of which are wrong. One temptation is to start changing your eating habits *now*, before you've planned out your system of mini-goals. This is likely to prove a haphazard and disappointing task because you won't have *easy* and *enjoyable* mini-goals set. You won't be able to clearly see how the changes you are making will fit into the overall scheme of things until you've written down your lists of mini-goals for changing sugar, fat, salt and fibre intake. So, don't try to start making improvements until you have properly organized yourself.

Apart from the temptation to get started before you are really ready, there is another, perhaps worse, temptation. You know you'll have your diary and be ready to start relatively soon. So you decide to make the most of the present time to have an enormous blow out; you eat as much high fat, high sugar, and salty food as you can possibly manage. Now, if a week from now, you were going to start a very rigid diet, or totally change your eating habits straight away, then this binge on the 'forbidden' foods would be quite understandable. It's very human to react to the possibility of deprivation by 'stoking up' in readiness. Many people, who go on strict diets with very limited food intake, binge before they start. It is often the case that they also binge after they finish their diets, which is why so many women never succeed in controlling their weight. However, when you start your regime about a week from now, you will be making very tiny changes to your normal food intake. You'll hardly notice the difference. And we don't want you to go hungry either. So there is no need to stuff yourself with food to prepare for an ordeal, because there won't be one! You're going to enjoy the changes you will be making.

However, the few days before you start *can* be very useful indeed. During this period don't change your normal eating pattern at all. This is an excellent time to get a clear idea of your present food habits. Before you can begin to change habits you first need to know exactly what those habits are. By accurately recording your food and drink intake for a few days, you obtain a 'baseline' of your behaviour. That is, you have a base, from which you can later work out a clear progression of mini-goals to your ultimate goals. Whilst obtaining your baseline, it is essential that you eat your usual food. Don't make *any* changes at all.

We are, of course, assuming that the few days before you start are typical days. If it happens to be Christmas, when you always eat differently, or if you are going on holiday where you will be eating different and exotic foods, then this obviously won't make a very good baseline. You can either wait until these unusual occasions have passed, and then start to record your typical food intake for a few days, *or* you can rely on memory to write down what your normal eating behaviour is like. Be careful here, though; memory can be notoriously unreliable!

When you are recording your normal daily intake, please make a note of all the following things:

1. the time the food or drink was consumed
2. the place the food or drink was consumed
3. the size of the portions of the food or drink
4. anything added to the food or drink (for example, salt in cooking or at the table; sugar in drinks or on cereal; butter on vegetables; salad cream on salad)
5. how hungry you were before you began to eat any meal or snack.

When you have a clear idea of your normal eating behaviour, try to decide on exactly what changes need to be made. You will probably find it easier to control your eating if you restrict yourself to a set number of meals and snacks each day. Some people also find that it helps if they restrict the places that they eat in the home. For example, you might choose to eat only in the kitchen or dining room, never in the lounge. If you have tempting food, such as chocolates, scattered around (in your handbag, in the lounge, in the kitchen, and so on) you will be constantly fighting temptation. Keep food in one place. If it's all in the kitchen it's less easy to find yourself nibbling at food without thinking about it. When you look at your baseline record, note how often you ate without feeling any real need to do so. These occasions will need to be cut down.

You will also need to work out your lists of mini-goals. Here is an example of how to make up lists of mini-goals. The woman in this example has recorded her eating behaviour for a week and her baseline reveals the following. She has three main meals a day, plus she nibbles at food (a chocolate here, a biscuit there) at least five or six times throughout the day. She has two spoons of sugar in each drink of tea or coffee. She likes sweet things generally, particularly biscuits, and she often has a sweet dessert after main meals. This woman uses plenty of butter, spreading it thickly on bread and adding a generous portion to vegetables. She uses lard or dripping rather than vegetable oil to cook with. She has fried food four or five times a week. She often has meat (about four or five times a week), and this is nearly always in the form of meat pies. She doesn't very often have fish or chicken (maybe once a week). She drinks ordinary milk, has about 1 lb (0.45 kg) of cheese a week, and between ten and twelve eggs. She uses plenty of salt in her cooking and adds a generous amount at the table. She eats white bread, no wholegrain breakfast cereals, and few vegetables. She eats fresh fruit about three times a week.

This woman looks at her baseline behaviour and then carefully works out her lists of mini-goals, making certain that she chooses to start with the changes which are easiest for her. She decides her eating pattern will be three meals a day, plus one snack mid-morning, one snack mid-afternoon, and a light supper. She won't eat between these six eating occasions. Her lists of mini-goals might look something like this:

*mini-goals for reducing sugar*
1. only 1 spoon of sugar in each tea or coffee
2. no sweet dessert with lunch
3. just one biscuit mid-morning and mid-afternoon (instead of the usual two or three!)
4. bake sugar-free biscuits. Have one mid-morning and one mid-afternoon.
5. no sugar in tea or coffee
6. have a sweet dessert after dinner only twice a week
7. buy low sugar jam as a substitute for ordinary jam
8. don't have anything sweet at supper time

*mini-goals for reducing fat*
1. try a low fat spread instead of butter
2. have fried food only once a week
3. buy sunflower oil rather than lard
4. try skimmed or semi-skimmed milk
5. cut the meat pies to twice a week
6. have lean meat instead of meat pies
7. have fish or chicken three times a week
8. use only a scrape of low fat spread on bread, and only a tiny amount on cooked vegetables
9. have a maximum of six eggs a week. No more than two eggs at any one meal
10. have skimmed milk or yogurt sometimes instead of cheese

*mini-goals for reducing salt*
1. use only about half the usual amount in cooking

2. use about half the amount of salt at table
3. buy potassium salt instead of table salt
4. stop eating salted foods (such as salted crisps and nuts)
5. use no salt in cooking

*mini-goals for increasing fibre intake*
1. eat more vegetables. Have pulses at least four times a week
2. eat more fruit (at least one piece a day)
3. try wholemeal bread for 2 days of the week
4. have a meal with wholegrain rice or pasta twice a week
5. have wholemeal bread all the time instead of white bread
6. try wholegrain cereal for breakfast.

This woman would start off with mini-goal 1 for sugar, fat, salt and fibre during week 1. In week 2, if she was successful with all of them, she would continue with what she was doing in week 1, plus she should go on to mini-goal no.2 for sugar, fat, salt and fibre. If she carries on like this, doing just that little bit more each week, by week 10 all the mini-goals will have been accomplished.

You'll note that it isn't necessary to have the same number of mini-goals for each thing you are trying to change. The harder it is for you to do something, the more steps (mini-goals) you need to break it into. Much better to have lots of tiny, easy steps than a few big ones. Of course, this means you'll probably achieve all your mini-goals for some things faster than others. The woman in our example achieved all her mini-goals for salt by week 5, all her mini-goals for fibre by week 6, all her mini-goals for sugar by week 8, and all her mini-goals for fat by week 10.

Every woman will have her own particular eating habits. People vary in the steps they find easiest to take. Consequently, your own individual lists of mini-goals will not be like anybody else's. It's entirely up to you to find the easiest path to success by making up lists of mini-goals that you feel confident you can achieve.

**How to achieve lasting success**
You may need to review your progress every now and again. For example, if you achieve all your mini-goals, you may be fine for a while, but then you may have extra difficulties which need to be tackled. For example, if you go away on holiday, you have less

control of your food and the way it is cooked. This doesn't matter. Enjoy the change, but remember, this is no time for gluttony. You won't properly enjoy your food unless you are hungry when you sit down to eat, so restrain yourself from just eating for the sake of it. Enjoy your food, eat until you are satisfied, then stop. Then you won't get fat. But it could be that after the holiday you find it difficult to revert back to your low sugar, low salt, low fat, high fibre food regime. If this is so, you might like to take 2 or 3 weeks to get back into it again. Make out some very short lists of mini-goals to get yourself readjusted.

Another time that you may need to review your progress is after the first trimester of the pregnancy. It could well be that you started your health programme early in the pregnancy, when you were occasionally suffering from feelings of sickness and therefore not wanting to eat a great deal. Under these conditions it was probably very easy to keep to all your mini-goals. However, when the sickness goes at about week 13, your appetite may return with a vengeance! If, by week 15 or 16, you realize that you have started to lose control (for example, eating too many sugary and fatty foods), you must rethink your plans. Look back at the section on food cravings at the end of Chapter 4. Remind yourself about how to deal with such cravings. Remember that it is very important to differentiate between a healthy drive to eat nutritious foods, and a yearn for lots of sugary foods which are low in essential nutrients. You do not need extra sugar. But are you actually eating enough good nutritious food at meals? Perhaps you should follow some of the planned menus we gave you in Chapter 4. What you may well need to do is take another baseline and work out some mini-goals again. For example, let us imagine it is now week 17 of the pregnancy. During week 16 you didn't keep to all of your mini-goals. So, what you must do is keep an accurate daily record of your food and drink habits during week 17 and get a fresh baseline. Don't try to be extra good during this week, just eat in as normal a way as possible. Then make out a whole new list of mini-goals for sugar, fat, salt and fibre. You'll probably find, this second time around, that it is much easier to introduce healthy behaviour change, and that you don't actually need so many mini-goals in your lists as you did the first time.

Never be frightened of failure. If you find that you are not keeping to your targets, this doesn't mean you are an inferior human being with no will-power! What it *does* mean is that, in all probability, various things are happening (like, it's Christmas; or you get invited out to dinner more often; or you're on holiday; or you're just bored with waiting for the baby to be born), and these events make your goals harder to maintain. This isn't a sign that you should abandon everything. It's a sign that you should think more carefully than ever about the best ways to tackle your problems. Rather than making out fresh lists of mini-goals, perhaps you ought to consider being a little extra kind to yourself, and allowing yourself one or two extra treats for a week or two. Never let yourself get to the state where you feel miserable or deprived. You'll only overcompensate and have a binge. It's much better to plan some special treats and remain in control.

**Your daily weight: what does it mean?**

We have recommended that you weigh each day, and we explained in Chapter 6 just how this should help you get in tune with the reasons why your weight changes. For example, a *sudden* increase of about 3 lb (1.4 kg) is most likely to mean that you've eaten a salty meal and are retaining water, or that you are constipated, rather than that you have gained 3 lb (1.4 kg) of body fat. Such a fast increase should be followed by a fast decrease when the problem causing it has gone.

During the first trimester you should stay approximately the same weight. This does not mean that you actually will weigh exactly the same each day. Your weight might be a little up on one day and a little down the next. But if you look at your diary for a period of, say, a month, you should be able to see if there is a trend upwards or downwards. Here is an example of a woman's weight each day in weeks 6, 7, 8 and 9 of the first trimester:

| week 6 | st | lb | (kg) |
|--------|----|----|------|
| Mon | 9 | 6 | 59.9 |
| Tues | 9 | 7 | 60.3 |
| Wed | 9 | 6 | 59.9 |
| Thur | 9 | 6 | 59.9 |
| Fri | 9 | 7 | 60.3 |
| Sat | 9 | 6 | 59.9 |
| Sun | 9 | 6 | 59.9 |

*week* 7

| | | | |
|---|---|---|---|
| Mon | 9 | 5 | 59.4 |
| Tues | 9 | 6 | 59.9 |
| Wed | 9 | 6 | 59.9 |
| Thur | 9 | 6 | 59.9 |
| Fri | 9 | 6 | 59.9 |
| Sat | 9 | 5 | 59.4 |
| Sun | 9 | 5 | 59.4 |

*week* 8

| | | | |
|---|---|---|---|
| Mon | 9 | 5 | 59.4 |
| Tues | 9 | 5 | 59.4 |
| Wed | 9 | 8 | 60.8 |
| Thur | 9 | 6 | 59.9 |
| Fri | 9 | 5 | 59.4 |
| Sat | 9 | 5 | 59.4 |
| Sun | 9 | 5 | 59.4 |

*week* 9

| | | | |
|---|---|---|---|
| Mon | 9 | 5 | 59.4 |
| Tues | 9 | 4 | 59.0 |
| Wed | 9 | 5 | 59.4 |
| Thur | 9 | 4 | 59.0 |
| Fri | 9 | 4 | 59.0 |
| Sat | 9 | 4 | 59.0 |
| Sun | 9 | 4 | 59.0 |

You can see that there is a slight variation from day to day. However, by the end of week 9 there is a clear trend beginning to show. This woman's pattern of weight indicates that she has lost about 2 lb (0.9 kg) during the month. During week 6 she either weighed 9 st 6 lb (59.9 kg) or 9 st 7 lb (60.3 kg). By week 8 she weighed 9 st 5 lb (59.4 kg) on some days. And by week 9 she was 9 st 4 lb (59.0 kg) on most days.

A small loss in weight like this, during the first trimester, is very common. However, although the quantity (in terms of calorie value) of food may be a little less than needed, the quality of food (in terms of essential nutrients) should be maintained by eating plenty of proteins, vegetables and fruit. If there is a large loss in weight at *any* time during pregnancy, consult your doctor.

In the second and third trimesters you should gain about 1 lb

(0.45 kg) a week (until about week 37 or 38). Now, this doesn't mean the weight will go on evenly, at the rate of one seventh of a pound (64 gm) a day. A more typical pattern for a month in the second or third trimester (where 4 lb or 1.8 kg is gained) would look like this:

| week 20 | st | lb | (kg) |
|---|---|---|---|
| Mon | 9 | 10 | 61.7 |
| Tues | 9 | 10 | 61.7 |
| Wed | 9 | 12 | 62.6 |
| Thur | 9 | 11 | 62.1 |
| Fri | 9 | 11 | 62.1 |
| Sat | 9 | 10 | 61.7 |
| Sun | 9 | 11 | 62.1 |
| | | | |
| week 21 | | | |
| Mon | 9 | 11 | 62.1 |
| Tues | 9 | 12 | 62.6 |
| Wed | 9 | 11 | 62.1 |
| Thur | 9 | 11 | 62.1 |
| Fri | 9 | 11 | 62.1 |
| Sat | 9 | 12 | 62.6 |
| Sun | 9 | 12 | 62.6 |
| | | | |
| week 22 | | | |
| Mon | 9 | 12 | 62.6 |
| Tues | 9 | 12 | 62.6 |
| Wed | 10 | 0 | 63.5 |
| Thur | 9 | 13 | 63.0 |
| Fri | 9 | 13 | 63.0 |
| Sat | 9 | 13 | 63.0 |
| Sun | 9 | 13 | 63.0 |
| | | | |
| week 23 | | | |
| Mon | 10 | 0 | 63.5 |
| Tues | 10 | 0 | 63.5 |
| Wed | 10 | 1 | 64.0 |
| Thur | 10 | 0 | 63.5 |
| Fri | 10 | 0 | 63.5 |
| Sat | 10 | 0 | 63.5 |
| Sun | 10 | 0 | 63.5 |

You can see that this woman is 9 st 10 lb or 61.7 kg on some days in week 20. The sudden increase to 9 st 12 lb (62.6 kg) on the Wednesday of week 20 is most likely to be caused by a salty meal the evening before, or maybe she forgot to empty her bladder before she weighed (and she should therefore have been around 9 st 11 lb or (62.1 kg), or maybe she is a little constipated. However, by week 21 some pregnancy weight has been added. In week 21 she is not 9 st 10 lb (61.7 kg) on any day; she is 9 st 11 lb (62.1 kg) on four days, indicating a genuine increase in weight directly associated with the pregnancy. This trend clearly continues, so that by week 23 she is 10 st 0 lb (63.5 kg) on most days. It would appear that she has gained about 4 lb (1.8 kg) in 4 weeks, and this is just right.

How would she know if she was gaining too much weight? If she was putting on fat as well as direct pregnancy weight, then weeks 20-23 may have looked something like this:

| week 20 | st | lb | (kg) |
|---|---|---|---|
| Mon | 9 | 10 | 61.7 |
| Tues | 9 | 10 | 61.7 |
| Wed | 9 | 12 | 62.6 |
| Thur | 9 | 12 | 62.6 |
| Fri | 9 | 12 | 62.6 |
| Sat | 9 | 11 | 62.1 |
| Sun | 9 | 12 | 62.6 |
| week 21 | st | lb | (kg) |
| Mon | 9 | 12 | 62.6 |
| Tues | 9 | 13 | 63.0 |
| Wed | 10 | 0 | 63.5 |
| Thur | 10 | 0 | 63.5 |
| Fri | 9 | 12 | 62.6 |
| Sat | 10 | 0 | 63.5 |
| Sun | 10 | 0 | 63.5 |
| week 22 | | | |
| Mon | 10 | 0 | 63.5 |
| Tues | 10 | 1 | 64.0 |
| Wed | 10 | 0 | 63.5 |
| Thur | 10 | 2 | 64.4 |
| Fri | 10 | 1 | 64.0 |

| | | | |
|---|---|---|---|
| Sat | 10 | 1 | 64.0 |
| Sun | 10 | 2 | 64.4 |

*week 23*

| | | | |
|---|---|---|---|
| Mon | 10 | 2 | 64.4 |
| Tues | 10 | 2 | 64.4 |
| Wed | 10 | 1 | 64.0 |
| Thur | 10 | 3 | 64.9 |
| Fri | 10 | 3 | 64.9 |
| Sat | 10 | 3 | 64.9 |
| Sun | 10 | 3 | 64.9 |

You can see that she looks to have gained about 7 lb (3.2 kg) rather than 4 lb (1.8 kg) over the 4 weeks. Does an extra 3 lb (1.4 kg) matter? Well, if this month is the only time she does gain too much, it probably doesn't matter a great deal. If she gains 25 lb (11.4 kg) over the whole pregnancy, instead of 22 lb (10 kg) she has still done very well. But, if she continues to put on 3 lb (1.4 kg) too much every month, she will finish grossly, and even dangerously, overweight.

So, you can see that you should take action as soon as you realize you are putting on too much weight. There will probably be no need to wait for 4 weeks before you spot a trend in weight change. In the above example, it is obvious by the Wednesday or Thursday of week 21 that something is wrong. The woman in this example should therefore have taken corrective action then. Maybe she should have taken a calorie counting spotcheck (as we described in the last chapter). She has almost certainly been eating too much in week 20 and the beginning of week 21. So, as soon as she realized this (say, the Wednesday of week 21) she *should not* go on a low calorie diet or eat a lot less, but she *should* reduce her food intake very slightly to get herself back to the proper rate of weight gain.

It becomes easier with practice to spot trends in weight change. Rather than just looking at the figures in a diary, many people find it useful to plot weight on a graph. Whether your weight is going up, down, or staying the same, is then very easy to see. You should notice a very slight deviation from the correct course, and you'll be able to make the small, relatively easy changes necessary to keep yourself to target.

Please remember NEVER to deprive yourself of the foods we recommended in Chapter 4. Have all the protein foods (from plant and animal sources), fruit and vegetables, that you need to satisfy your appetite. If you do need to cut back on food to keep your weight gain to that which is medically recommended, try your best to have less of the very sugary foods. It will not harm you or the baby if you stop having things like cakes, biscuits, sweets, ice cream and sugar, and if you don't have sweet fizzy drinks.

# 8

# Getting The Exercise Right

As we have already outlined, weight control is a matter of achieving the right balance between the foods you take in and the energy you burn up. Exercise is a vital part of this balancing act. Not only does it enable you to obtain the right match between your intake and your output, it also has other benefits. The improvement in your muscles which results from exercise will give your body a firmer, healthier appearance, enabling you to maintain not only the weight you want but also the shape you want. In addition, exercise can do much to avoid the common problems of pregnancy, like backache, constipation and varicose veins. To obtain the most benefit from exercise, however, two things are necessary. First, it is necessary to match the level and kind of exercise to your own abilities. Second, it is necessary to match the level and kind of exercise to the stage of your pregnancy. In this chapter we aim to provide you with guidelines for doing both of these.

**How fit are you to start with?**
Obviously, before setting out on any exercise programme, it is helpful to know at least roughly how fit you are to begin with. Many medical experts believe that the pattern of exercise in pregnancy depends a lot on what kind of exercise you're normally used to; most people, with little or no exercise background, will need to increase their level of exercise slightly, whilst those who are normally highly trained athletes will probably be best taking things a little easier than they normally do.

Scientists have developed many complicated methods of

assessing fitness. For our purposes, however, all we need is a rough way of judging approximately how fit you are. We can think of people as falling into one of five broad categories:

1. the very unfit in poor health
2. those who aren't as fit as they could be but are in generally good health
3. those who are both healthy and a little fitter than average
4. the very fit living a healthy life style, and
5. top competitive athletes

In this chapter we will be offering little advice to those in groups 1 and 5. These two extremes each require more careful consideration than can be given in a book of this nature. Group 1 will need to consult carefully with their doctors in order to decide what, if any, exercise they're capable of without risk. At the opposite extreme, group 5 will almost certainly want to consult their coaches and the national medical officers of their sport before deciding on an appropriate level of exercise. Even for these two groups, however, it may be beneficial to read through this chapter so as to obtain a basis which they can adapt, with suitable guidance, for their own particular needs.

For other women we will be giving methods of obtaining a rough idea of whether you're in group 2, 3 or 4 and then some approaches to exercise appropriate to each stage. The suggestions we give for exercise will need to be interpreted using the assessment of your own fitness together with a little common sense. For example, if you're in group 2 you may wish to build up your exercise gradually at this stage, whilst if in group 4, you may be able to do rather more than we suggest. You should be ready to adjust your level of exercise as you're going along; if you decide you're only a group 2 person but then find some of the exercises too easy, you can do a little more on those particular ones. Because our categories are only approximate, you may well find you're like a group 2 person for some exercises but group 4 for others. However, you shouldn't make any sudden increases in the exercise routine you adopt; some of the things we suggest might seem too easy to start with, but remember you'll be doing some of them over a period of several months, and if you start at too difficult a level you might find it hard to keep up.

So how do you decide which group you're in? One of the simplest ways of assessing your fitness is to decide how overweight you are. You will often see tables published which tell you your ideal weight for someone your height. To use these properly, you need to know if you're a person of small, medium or large frame. One way to judge this is to measure around the narrowest part of your wrist. If it is less than 5.5 in (14 cm), you are a small frame. If it is over 6.5 in (15.5 cm) you are a large frame. Anything in between is medium. These estimates can make a big difference to your ideal weight. For example, a 5-foot (152.5 cm) woman, aged 25, should weigh between 7 st 4 lb (46.5 kg) and 7 st 12 lb (50 kg) if she is small frame, but between 8 st 3 lb (52 kg) and 9 st 4 lb (59 kg) if she is large frame. This means that it's possible for two women to have the same height and weight (say 5 feet tall and 8 stone) and for one to be underweight, if she's large frame, and the other overweight, if she's small frame.

If you don't have suitable tables available to read off the correct weight for your height, an approximation can easily be made with the help of a pocket calculator. Take your weight in kg (you can obtain this by multiplying your weight in pounds by 0.45). Measure your height, without shoes, in metres (this is your height in inches multiplied by 0.0254). Divide your weight in kg by your height in metres, then divide the answer by your height in metres once more. This measure (weight divided by height squared) should be similar for similar framed women whatever their height. Your answer should be between 19 and 21 for a small frame, and 20 and 22.5 for a medium frame, and 21.5 and 24.5 for a large frame. If the answer you obtain is more than 4 over the upper limit for your frame, you are very overweight.

This gives us a start on deciding which group you fall into. To decide on your group, answer the following questions:

(i)    Are you very overweight?          YES/NO
(ii)   Do you smoke?                       YES/NO
(iii)  Are you over 30?                    YES/NO

If you answered YES to all three then you are in group 1 and should definitely not exercise without consulting your doctor. You should also put yourself in group 1 if at any time your resting blood pressure is found to be high. And if you have had a previous miscarriage you should put yourself in group 1. Remember group 1 women should NOT exercise without first consulting their doctor.

If you are not in group 1 you should be able to find a safe level of exercise which will help you control your weight and will leave both you and your baby healthy. If you represent your country, county or area in any sport, at national or international level, you should regard yourself as being in group 5. Women in this group (Olympic athletes, international swimmers, runners etc.) will probably ease back a little on their training during pregnancy. However, future sporting careers may be at stake, and to decide how much exercise to do, it will be necessary to work out a detailed individual programme with your coach.

Most of you, however, will be neither group 1 nor group 5. This leaves us with groups 2, 3 and 4. To see if you fall into group 2, answer the following questions:

(i)   Is your weight within acceptable limits?   YES/NO
(ii)  Do you play any sports regularly?   YES/NO
(iii) Do you do any other exercise regularly?   YES/NO
      (e.g. jogging, aerobics, dance class)
(iv)  Do you practise any form of yoga?   YES/NO
(v)   Are you a non-smoker?   YES/NO
(vi)  Is your pulse, when relaxed, over 95 beats YES/NO
      per minute? (Only answer this if you're
      still in the first 6 weeks of your pregnancy)

You shouldn't answer question (vi) unless you're still in the first 6 weeks of your pregnancy, as pregnancy itself will affect your pulse. If, however, you know what your resting pulse was before you became pregnant, you can use that figure.

If you answered NO to three or more questions (or to two or more if you missed out question (vi)), you should regard yourself as group 2 – not as fit as you could be but in generally good health. Otherwise you are in groups 3 or 4. To decide which, answer the following:

(i)   Do you take some specific exercise most
      days?   YES/NO
(ii)  Do you play any sport competitively?   YES/NO
(iii) Are you a non-smoker?   YES/NO

(iv) Are you under 25 and the right weight? YES/NO

(v) Is your pulse, when relaxed, below 65
beats per minute? (Only answer this if
you're still in the first 6 weeks of your
pregnancy)         YES/NO

If you answered NO to three or more questions (or two or more if you didn't answer question (v)), it's probably best to think of yourself in group 3 – healthy and a little fitter than average. If you answered YES to three or more questions, put yourself in group 4. You're obviously in good condition – something of a keep-fit enthusiast perhaps?

Now that you know roughly your level of fitness you have a basis for doing the kinds of exercise we describe in the rest of the chapter. Where we give a specific amount or number of exercises. this should be within the capabilities of group 3 unless we say otherwise. Group 2 should also be able to do the amount suggested, but may need to build up to it over a few weeks. Group 4 on the other hand will probably be able to start at the level suggested and may be able to do rather more if it seems too easy.

## Exercises for pregnancy

We realize that the majority of women who read this book will already be pregnant. Nevertheless, those of you who are planning a pregnancy, rather than pregnant already, can start to take useful steps to prepare for pregnancy. The rest of you, already pregnant, can read quickly through the next paragraph and go on to the next where we provide guidelines for exercise during pregnancy.

The time when you're planning pregnancy, rather than actually pregnant, is a good time to develop the right exercise habits. Exactly what kind of exercise you do is to some extent up to you – but if possible, it should be fun. It's a good idea to think about the kinds of exercise you'll be able to continue during your pregnancy – so if you normally take your exercise doing sports like squash or judo, this may be a time to make a change to something like swimming or jogging.

To exercise most effectively in pregnancy involves three types of activity: some specific exercises which are useful for pregnant women; general forms of exercise; and modifications of normal day-to-day activities. Each of these is quite simple.

*Specific exercises of value in pregnancy*
The specific exercises we describe are designed to help with the particular problems of pregnancy. Each is useful, although it is important to match each of them to the stage of your pregnancy; we will give you advice on this later in the chapter. First, however, a description of the exercises themselves:

*Situps*: lie on your back on the floor with your knees slightly bent and your feet on the ground. It helps if you can persuade a partner to hold your feet on the ground. Clasp your hands behind your neck and try to lift your head and shoulders off the ground. Group 4 and some of group 3 should be able to sit up completely. Others may only be able to lift head and shoulders a few inches. Once you've raised your head and shoulders as much as possible, lower yourself gently to the ground and repeat. You should aim to be able to do this five to ten times in any session.

For those of you who find it difficult to sit up completely, you can give yourselves a start by placing a number of cushions under your head and shoulders to begin with. Then as you get better and better you can gradually use fewer and fewer cushions.

Finally, with respect to situps, watch out for a couple of points. When lowering yourself to the ground, do so slowly – don't just drop down. Apart from the risk of banging your head on the floor, you miss half of the exercise if you don't do the work of lowering yourself slowly. Also make sure that you keep your knees bent throughout the exercise; in the past, situps were often done with the legs held straight, but more recently it has become clear that this puts excessive strain on the back and can lead to injury – so if anyone says you should have your legs straight, they're out of date. Situps are good for both abdominal and back muscles, making it easier to carry your baby, reducing the risk of back problems, and helping you regain your shape quickly after the birth.

*Hyperextensions*: in a way these are the opposite of situps. Lie face down on the floor with a partner holding your feet down. Clasp your hands behind your neck and raise your head gently off the ground by arching your back. Lower yourself slowly. Each part of the movement should be slow and gentle, lasting about 3 seconds. Again, you should aim to do at least ten in any one session.

Hyperextensions are a good way of strengthening the muscles in your back, and thereby reducing the risk of later problems. Obviously, they are to be done relatively early in your pregnancy, before your change of shape makes them impractical.

*Knee bends*: stand with your back to the wall, your heels together against the skirting and your big toes about 8 or 9 in (20 cm) apart, so that your feet are pointing away from each other at an angle of about 90 degrees. Slowly bend your legs, keeping your back and shoulders flat against the wall. Your knees should point in the same direction as your toes. As you bend your legs further you will reach a point where your heels start to come off the ground. When you reach this point you should slowly straighten your legs again. Once your legs are straight, continue the movement so that you come up on your toes; pause briefly then return to your starting position. These exercises will help strengthen your legs and will assist in developing good posture. Remember to do the exercises slowly. You should aim to be able to do twenty-five or more in a single session.

*Toe touches*: sit on the ground with your feet as wide apart as is comfortable and your toes pointing to the ceiling. Reach your arms high in the air but without hunching your shoulders. This should give your body a feeling of 'lifting' out of the ground. Keeping your arms stretched and maintaining the lifting feeling, slowly reach your left hand to your left foot, rise again, then reach your right hand to your right foot and return to the starting position. Then repeat the exercise taking your left hand to your right foot and your right hand to your left foot.

It's unlikely that you'll actually be able to reach your toes, even if you're in groups 3 or 4 unless you've been involved in some activity which places a high premium on suppleness (e.g. yoga, karate, contemporary dance). Don't force the movement but keep it gentle, going only as far as you can comfortably, then rising again. Try to keep your legs fairly straight but don't force them into a rigid position – a slight bend at the knees is quite acceptable. This exercise is extremely good for strengthening the muscles in the back and thereby avoiding backache. It is, however, quite difficult and you should start off doing only two or three per session and building up to six or eight.

*Breathing*: for each of the exercises we've just described, it's worth paying a little attention to breathing patterns. At all times your breathing should be slow and calm. Most of the exercises have an easier and harder part. In situps, for example, the return to lying flat is easier than the actual sitting up, because you have gravity to help you. When doing your exercises try to take one slow, continuous breath IN during the easy part, then a slow continuous breath OUT during the harder part. So, for example, during the hyperextensions you should breathe OUT to the count of three when lifting your head, then IN to the count of three when lowering it again. This may take a little getting used to at first, but if you concentrate it will soon become automatic.

*Relaxation*: as we mentioned in Chapter 5, relaxation is an important part of exercise. Full instructions on relaxation training would almost fill a book by themselves. However, there are some basic procedures which can be a big help in learning to relax.

Perhaps the most simple of these is to set aside time for relaxing. The exercises we've just described shouldn't take more than 15 or 20 minutes to do. If you then set aside a further 25 or 30 minutes for relaxation you can have completed all you need to do some days in one three-quarter of an hour period. Besides setting aside time, try to set aside a place. Probably the most obvious is a bedroom, but a comfortable chair may be equally good or better if you prefer. Do not have any bright lights on, and try to be at least a little sheltered from surrounding noises.

To increase your relaxation you should either lie on your back, hands resting lightly by your side or on your body. If you're sitting in a chair, you should sit comfortably, with your hands either by your side or resting in your lap. Slowly close your eyes and concentrate on breathing (you might find it helpful to have someone read these instructions to you whilst you practice with your eyes closed). Breathe in slowly, pause, then breathe out slowly, pause, and continue like this until the pattern of breathing becomes automatic and natural.

Try to picture in your imagination the kind of situation in which you feel really relaxed – for example, lying on the beach in the warm sunshine. Picture yourself in this kind of situation. Imagine you can feel the warmth of the sun on your skin, that you can hear the soft sound of the sea in the distance. All the time keep breathing slowly and steadily. This procedure can lead by itself to a pleasant and light state of relaxation.

Deeper levels of relaxation can be obtained by concentrating on individual muscles. The details of such procedures would take too long to go into, but you may like to try concentrating on muscles in your hands, imagining them feeling really heavy, and then repeating the procedure for other major muscles in your body. You might, for example, start with your hands, then your arms, shoulders, neck and legs. By concentrating at all times on the sensations produced by imagining the feeling of heaviness, you should be able to induce a state of deep relaxation. For a really deep state of relaxation you can combine the feeling of heaviness with tensing of the muscles, holding the tension for a few seconds, and then suddenly letting the tension go. By doing this with the muscles of your arms, neck, body and legs, it's possible to obtain a very deep state of relaxation. To help with these kinds of procedure, many health shops and the like sell cassette tapes which give instructions for relaxation procedures.

However deeply you go into the relaxation, you should finish the session as gently as you started. Don't set an alarm clock to suddenly bring you back to full alertness. Rather start to feel the sensations in your muscles again, starting to move them slightly and slowly, opening your eyes and only standing up again when you've had a little time to re-orient yourself to your normal state.

By using relaxation procedures in this way you will not only be able to obtain the benefits of a period of time spent totally relaxed, but will also find yourself more able to relax at other times. When life is becoming a little stressful, or you feel yourself becoming a little tense, your practice at relaxing will enable you to relax more easily and avoid many of the harmful effects of stress.

You'll perhaps find it easiest to combine the various exercises we described earlier (situps, hyperextensions etc.) with the relaxation as a single session. How often you do the exercises, and which ones you do, will depend both on how fit you are and what stage of your pregnancy you're in. Later in the chapter we'll have a little to say about linking the exercises to your stage of pregnancy.

First, however, it's worth thinking a little about the more general activities which might be used to contribute to your exercise programme in pregnancy.

*General activities for exercise in pregnancy*
Obviously, many of you will at some time in your lives have thought about or participated in activities which provide useful exercise. You may have played competitive sports, practised yoga, taken ballet classes or something similar. Many of these can be of great value in pregnancy if approached appropriately. In general, it is probably best to look to activities which provide fairly rhythmic, gentle actions and avoid violent or highly vigorous actions. Thus, steady jogging is better than a series of short sprints. If you play games like tennis or badminton, try to avoid doing so competitively; instead, ask your partner to play co-operatively, making it easy for you to reach the return shots. Many exercises are suitable for pregnant women. Below we comment on some of the more commonly recommended ones and how you might go about these. If you wish to do some other form of exercise, instead or as well as the ones below, the essential principles are that you should try to remain relaxed whilst doing them, that you should not attempt to push yourself too hard, and that you should avoid pain.

*Running*: done properly, running can be one of the most valuable forms of exercise during pregnancy. If you are going to run during pregnancy it is essential that you follow the guidelines we gave you in Chapter 5 for obtaining a suitable pair of training shoes. When you go out running don't worry too much about the speed you run at; try to settle into a relaxed, easy rhythm. If you're running correctly you should find that you are breathing a little more heavily than normal but that you can still maintain a conversation (try running with a partner to check this). Many people find it difficult to relax whilst running. It helps if you take relatively short strides and lean your body slightly forward. If your neck and shoulders feel tense you should consciously try to make the back of your neck feel longer, without the front being shorter (see below under 'posture'). You may also find that resting the tip of your index finger lightly against the tip of your thumb helps to relax you.

Just as you shouldn't worry about how fast you run, neither should you worry about how far. Indeed, for those of you in groups 2 and 3 it's probably best to concentrate on how many minutes you can keep running rather than how many miles. A woman in group 3 should be able to jog gently along for about 5 to 6 minutes with a little practice; group 2 women might need a few sessions to build up to this from about 2 to 3 minutes per session. Both groups should aim to be able to jog along for at least 10 minutes and possibly up to quarter of an hour. Don't, however, try to do this every day; every 2 days is probably the most useful frequency as this gives the intervening day to recover. Alternatively, you might aim to go jogging three times a week, perhaps on Sundays, Tuesdays and Thursdays. That way you obtain a day's rest after each of the first two with an extra day's rest after every third session.

For a couple of days after your first attempts you may feel some stiffness in your muscles – particularly in your legs but possibly also in your back and shoulders. Muscular stiffness in the legs is best dealt with by walking around, and if you can persuade yourself to go out for your next scheduled run, this too will help get rid of the stiffness. A slight stiffness in back and shoulders can be dealt with in the same way, with a little more care taken to relax on the run. Severe stiffness in your back or shoulders, however, should probably be given a few days' rest before starting again a little more gently.

Finally, a brief word about running for women in group 4. Many of you will have some experience of running, either as a sport in itself or as a training for some other sport. If you are an experienced runner you may well want to do more than suggested for the group 2 and group 3 women. You're also probably more used to dealing in miles or km than in minutes. If you are in this group, it's still worth keeping your distance down to a reasonable level. Aim to do not more than 4 miles (6.5 km) in any one run, and no more than four runs per week. Your weekly mileage should therefore be no more than 16 miles (26 km) and a total distance of 12 to 13 miles (19 to 21 km) per week is quite adequate. As with groups 2 and 3, it is important to stay relaxed and keep the running down to a gentle pace.

*Swimming*: like running, swimming is often recommended as a suitable exercise during pregnancy. Indeed, it has the advantage over running that it does not involve repeated striking of the feet on the ground which may occasionally lead to injury in runners who try to do too much or who wear shoes which are totally unsuitable. A further advantage is that the only clothing needed for swimming is usually already in your possession. Swimming has its disadvantages, however. It will usually involve more time. Not only does the equivalent amount of swimming involve longer sessions than running, but to this is added (for most of us) the need to travel to and from the pool etc. In some areas local authorities have organized special sessions for pregnant women where suitable exercises can be performed under the guidance of a trained teacher. If such sessions are available in your area, it is well worth making the effort to go along to them. You can find out if such sessions are available by telephoning your local council.

If, however, you are going to determine your own level of exercise in the swimming pool, it's worth following a few guidelines. As with running, it's important to remain relaxed whilst swimming, so don't force yourself to swim as hard as possible. Rather, you should aim to travel smoothly and gently through the water; breaststroke is probably the most suitable of strokes. Don't go so fast or so far that you're completely out of breath, but rather so that you're breathing just a little bit more heavily than normal. Take plenty of rests during the session – if possible, swim fairly close to the edge of the pool so that you can stop and hold on to the edge if you start to tire.

Like running, those of you in group 2 and group 3 will be best advised to aim for a total amount of time swimming rather than any particular distance. Try to aim for your total swimming time (excluding the break for rests) to be between 15 and 20 minutes. You will probably need to build up to this, however, starting at about 5 or 6 minutes. If you're needing frequent rest breaks to start with, be careful not to get too cold. Many people find that swimming gives them quite an appetite. Treat this with a little caution. A cup of hot tea or coffee after swimming is not a bad idea, but try to wait at least a quarter of an hour after having this (preferably half an hour) before eating. By then your appetite may have settled a little and you'll be less likely to overeat. As with running, do no more than a session every alternate day.

Group 4 women may have more experience of swimming, and certainly those of you who have been competitive swimmers may feel that the guidelines for groups 2 and 3 are a little too easy. Remember, however, that your swimming technique may be more efficient than most of the group 2 and group 3 women, and that you'll therefore cover more distance during the same amount of time. Increase the total a little if you wish, but it's probably best to do no more than half an hour's swimming in any one session, and no more than four sessions per week.

*Aerobics, dance and 'keep fit'*: these and similar classes are now available in many areas, and quite a few of you reading this book may have been regular attenders at such classes before you became pregnant. In principle, it's quite possible to continue such classes throughout your pregnancy, as long as a few simple guidelines are followed. The most important of these is to let your teacher know right away that you're pregnant. Some of the exercises may need some adaptation for you and you should follow the advice of a qualified teacher.

Classes like these make a number of different demands on the body. Firstly, they work the muscles, providing a steady rhythmic sequence which gives muscle tone and improves aerobic capacity (endurance). Before you were pregnant you may have become quite breathless during some sessions; during your pregnancy it's probably best to ease back a little, so that doing the class makes you breathe a little harder than usual but not much. If you start to become very breathless, stop and rest for a few minutes.

The second main demand classes like these make is on your suppleness. The movements may extend the range of a number of joints and lead you to become more flexible. However, we've already seen that pregnancy itself can increase your flexibility. Indeed, there's a danger during pregnancy that flexibility can become excessive with muscles not being able to keep up with the increased range of movement. Whilst you're pregnant, therefore, you should perform the various movements well within the range of your abilities. If you were doing the class before you became pregnant, resist the temptation to exploit the softness of tendons to extend your range of movement. Rather, you should keep in mind the amount you could do prior to your pregnancy, and do no more than this. Your range of movement in joints should not, as far as these classes are concerned, increase during pregnancy.

As a final note on these types of class, you should use a little caution where activities like running and jumping are concerned. Just a little of these is unlikely to do any harm, but remember that usually these classes are either taken barefoot or with only light shoes. Your feet will therefore not obtain the necessary support, and too much running or jumping may carry the risk of fallen arches whilst your tendons and ligaments are softened by pregnancy.

*Yoga*: various forms of yoga have become popular in recent years. Many of the comments we made about aerobics, dance and keep fit classes also apply to yoga. In particular, it is important that when you're pregnant you avoid any attempt to make your joints increase in range or suppleness. Yoga can often provide a good way of relaxing and avoiding day-to-day stresses. Many of the positions, however, are designed to stretch tendons in their normal state; during pregnancy the same exercises may cause overstretching. Again, the secret is to keep well within your normal capabilities. If a full lotus position is difficult, for example, stick to a half-lotus during pregnancy. You should at best only aim to maintain your flexibility during pregnancy, not to increase it.

On the positive side, many yoga exercises provide a good way of strengthening the back muscles. As long as these are not attempted with too much effort, yoga can have much to offer, particularly in avoiding later back problems. Yoga will not, however, do much to increase aerobic capacity. Remember, therefore, that if you are doing yoga this should be supplemented with some other form of exercise which will make your heart and lungs work a little harder than normal.

*Cycling*: in many ways this is close to being an ideal form of exercise for pregnant women. It can provide aerobic exercise without the shock of pounding the roads that running involves. Unlike swimming (for most of us), it involves getting out into the fresh air and, importantly, sunlight. Remember that even a little sunlight on a winter's day can do much to help provide your body's needs of vitamin D.

In practice, cycling is not always as good as it could be. Unless you're very confident on a bicycle there's always the possibility that whilst you're pregnant you'll be extra worried about keeping your balance. Such worry may make it difficult to relax. For many women cycling will involve main roads and traffic, the fumes of which are not good for you or your baby. In addition, there is always the risk of accidents when riding in traffic. However, for the woman who is used to cycling and who has quiet country roads to go along, cycling can be heartily recommended.

The problem of traffic and fumes can be avoided by using a stationary exercise bicycle instead of a real one. Usually, however, you'll be using such a machine indoors, where of course you won't be getting the fresh air or sunshine. Nevertheless, an exercise bicycle does provide a way of obtaining aerobic exercise in safety and relative comfort. If you are using such a device, adopt much the same guidelines as for swimming. Stay relaxed, work at a rate which causes you to breathe just a little more heavily than normal, and rest if you start to get tired. Like swimming, aim to build up to 15 or 20 minutes of easy pedalling – perhaps whilst watching your favourite TV programme?

One word of warning about exercise bicycles. There are a number of cheap models on the market which are likely to do more harm than good. Do try out a bicycle before buying one. It should be stable, with no risk of toppling sideways or backwards, and should have a smooth pedalling motion when in use. Avoid anything on which the pedal action is the least bit jerky. This will mean that to obtain a suitable bicycle you may have to spend over three times the price of the cheapest types, but the extra money is well spent.

Of course, as we mentioned earlier, there are many other exercises you can do besides the ones we've mentioned (running, swimming, keep fit classes, yoga and cycling). Reading through the guidelines we've given should provide you with a basis on which to design your own programme if you have a particular favourite pastime we haven't mentioned. Your chosen method, or methods of exercise should, if possible, involve some sustained level of activity which causes you to breathe just a little harder than normal. It should not place extra demands on suppleness, and it should involve at least some outdoor activity. Obviously, it will be easier to achieve all of these if you use a combination of activities. Remember to do this sensibly. If you've been running regularly and decide to do some swimming, introduce the swimming instead of, not as well as one of your normal running sessions. Exercise is important during pregnancy, but to do you good, it must be combined with rest and relaxation.

*Improvements in day-to-day activities*
Besides the kinds of specific exercise described above, there are a number of ways in which day-to-day activities can be modified to provide benefit in pregnancy. There are several things you could do as you go about your normal activities. In particular, you might consider the following:

*Walk, don't ride*: when going a fairly short distance, for example down to the shops, think first about whether you might walk rather than drive or catch a bus. Obviously, this will depend on such things as how far it is, how much you have to carry and how you're feeling at the time. By walking rather than riding you take a little more exercise and obtain the benefits of daylight and fresh air. You may feel up to walking a little more briskly than usual, which again will help increase your total amount of exercise.

*Watch your posture*: many of us, most of the time, do not have quite such good posture as we should. In the later stages of pregnancy posture may become even worse as your shape changes. Good posture, however, is not difficult to develop. In essence, good posture requires you to maintain a balanced, upright stance whilst at the same time staying relaxed. For example, when standing you should keep your weight evenly on both feet, your shoulders relaxed and your head held high. Try to imagine that all the individual bones in your spine are precisely balanced on top of each other. A good way to help relax is to remember to relax your hands – with your hands relaxed your arms and shoulders will usually follow suit. In addition, you can concentrate on the feeling of 'lengthening' your neck. If you imagine being gently lifted by someone taking hold of the hair on the crown of your head you can imagine the right sort of feeling – it should be as if the back of your neck is being lengthened without the front being shortened. Your shoulders should 'hang' relaxed, without slouching, and the whole feeling should be poised and comfortable.

*Don't stand still*: often during the day we do things which involve us standing in one place for fairly long periods of time. An example might be standing at the kitchen sink for 10 minutes or more to do the washing up. Standing still for a couple of minutes will do no harm at all. If you stand still for too long, however, this can impair your circulation and may lead to such problems as varicose veins.

One possible way round this is to keep your legs moving even if you yourself are standing still. Try walking on the spot for about 30 seconds, by bending first your right knee (lifting your right heel off the ground) then your left knee (lifting your left heel off the ground). If you continue this 'walking' for about half a minute, then rest for half a minute, then repeat the walking (and so on throughout the time you're standing there), the movement in your leg muscles will help the blood to circulate, reducing the strain on the veins in your legs and keeping them healthy.

*Lift carefully*: even when you're not pregnant incorrect lifting can lead to serious back problems. Back pain is one of the most common and at the same time one of the most difficult problems encountered by general practitioners. Often a major contributor to the problem has been the person's poor lifting technique. When picking things off the floor don't bend at the waist, keeping your legs almost straight. This puts far too much strain on the back. Rather, you should lift by keeping your back fairly straight and bending at the knees. You can then use the much stronger mucles of the legs to do the lifting and avoid straining your back.

The importance of good lifting technique can't be emphasized too strongly. Whilst it's important at all times, it is essential during pregnancy. The softening of tendons and ligaments whilst you're pregnant makes you particularly susceptible to pain and injury. A joint like the sacro-iliac joint, which joins the pelvic girdle to the spine, is rarely problematic for most women. However, during pregnancy the joint loosens, making the risk of back pain much higher unless care is taken. Similar difficulties arise in other parts of the back. Remember that if you develop back problems in pregnancy these won't necessarily go away later – some such problems will persist for years. You don't want to find that back pain means you're unable to pick up the beautiful baby you're going to have.

Thus, to summarize what we've said so far, exercise in pregnancy involves three different aspects. There are the specific exercises which are particularly helpful for you in pregnancy, more general exercises and slight modifications to your normal day-to-day activities to help avoid particular problems. As we mentioned earlier, your overall level of exercise in pregnancy will depend on how fit you are to start with. During your pregnancy, however, you will need to adapt your exercise to the different things going on in your body at different stages. We finish this chapter therefore with a few words on how to select your exercise according to the stage of your pregnancy.

## Matching exercise to your stage of pregnancy

Although your body goes through a large number of changes whilst you're pregnant, it's convenient as far as exercise planning is concerned to continue thinking in terms of the three trimesters. Each of these has its own specific characteristics which will affect both the amount and kind of exercise which is appropriate.

### The first trimester

During the first trimester of pregnancy many women report feeling tired and lethargic, and in consequence it may be difficult to motivate yourself to exercise. On the other hand it's also a time when you should give a great deal of thought to your physical activities. If you're fitter than average to start with, you may find that you can continue with sports like swimming and jogging, although you may not wish to do as much of these as before you were pregnant. Many of you, however, may feel that you're just too tired to do anything.

Rather than give in completely to this feeling, you may wish to compromise. If you don't feel up to it, leave the jogging and similar activities for a while. Instead, try to develop the habit of doing the kinds of specific exercises we described earlier (situps, hyperextensions etc.) It probably helps if you try to do these at the same time every day. If you decide to do them as soon as you get up, it's especially important that you shouldn't try too hard. During the night your body loses some of its suppleness, so don't try to force any of these exercises. If you remember to take care this way, first thing in the morning can be an excellent time to do the exercises. Try to do them, if possible, at least four times a week – though with these exercises at this stage there's no reason why you shouldn't do them every day.

One thing which is very important at this stage is to develop the relaxation habit. It might seem a little strange getting out of bed to do exercises only to follow them with going back to being relaxed – but it IS a good habit. Incidentally, there's no need always to precede your relaxation with the exercises. The relaxation can profitably be practised on its own as well, and you may wish to do this more than once a day. Again, it may be helpful to set aside a particular time of day to help the habit establish. Remember that you should regard relaxation as being at least as important as the more strenuous exercises.

Finally, it's worth remembering the various suggestions we made about day-to-day activities. If you feel particularly tired during this stage of pregnancy, you may not feel inclined to do very much walking about. Even so, be sure not to become totally inactive and sluggish – a brisk walk in fresh air may even make you feel better. The other aspects of day-to-day activities should depend less on your stage of pregnancy, and tired or not you should try to remember them. Try to develop a better posture during the first trimester, build up the habit of moving your legs when standing (or even sitting) still for any length of time. Most of all, be determined at this stage to break any bad lifting habits – always bend at the knees and try to keep your back upright.

*The second trimester*
During the second trimester you'll probably start to feel a lot better; indeed this is often a time when people describe the pregnant woman as 'blooming'. This can be a good time to change your exercise pattern. During the second trimester your body will be showing some substantial changes in shape, and this will affect the suitability of some of the specific exercises we suggested. You'll probably want to stop doing the hyperextensions, as lying

face down becomes less comfortable. You may also find the situps less and less comfortable. On the other hand, the toe-touching exercises may be quite comfortable throughout this stage, and it's probably a good idea to continue with the knee-bending exercise. Over all, you should use your own judgement throughout this period as to how your choice of basic exercises goes. Try to keep on doing as many as possible, but avoid strain or discomfort. The relaxation, of course, is well worth continuing, although if you've been relaxing in a chair it's not a bad idea at this stage to have some sessions lying on a bed, perhaps with a pillow under your feet to raise them a little.

Shaking off any feelings of tiredness during this period means, of course, that you can start to indulge in more general forms of exercise. Indeed, in one study of the effects of exercise the researchers particularly emphasized that the pregnant woman should make the most of feeling particularly well during the second trimester. Building up gradually on any of the activities we described earlier in the chapter (or a combination of them) can provide a good foundation for the later stages of pregnancy. Exercise which causes you to breathe just a little more heavily than normal is about the level you want. As with the specific exercises, remember that the exercise is only of value if combined with rest – so for these activities try to alternate exercise days with rest days if at all possible.

By this stage you should have built up the habit of conducting your normal daily activities in as healthy a way as possible. Walking may well be easier in this stage, and you may wish to go out for a walk purely for exercise, as well as the walking which is part of normal day-to-day life. Keeping your posture good, your leg muscles moving, and your lifting technique correct should become almost automatic. This stage of pregnancy is a chance to really prepare your body for the final months of your pregnancy – don't waste the opportunity.

*The third trimester*
By the start of the third trimester your weight will be around 12 lb (5.5 kg) above your normal weight. Throughout this final stage your weight will continue to increase, your shape will change more and more, and of course, exercise will become progressively more difficult.

This is a stage of gradually tapering off most of the exercise. The specific exercises probably don't need to be continued long into the third trimester (you'll have stopped the hyperextensions and probably the situps by now anyway). Exercises like jogging, swimming and the like can be continued for a while though you'll perhaps find it most useful to reduce gradually both the amount you do in each session and the number of sessions you do per week. By the time you're within 3 weeks of the expected delivery date you should have stopped these exercises altogether. Don't, however, stop suddenly. Plan in your diary how you're going to 'fade out' the activities, perhaps reducing to two sessions a week for a few weeks, then one session a week for a few more, and then perhaps missing out a whole week, having one more go, then stopping altogether until after the birth.

The points we made about day-to-day activities, however, will largely apply right up to the birth. You should try to keep moving as much as possible, although of course, walking any substantial distance will eventually become too tiring. Your posture should remain good, despite the shift forward in your balance because you're carrying the baby. If you've been doing the exercises this imbalance can be dealt with by your back muscles, which should be nice and strong by now. Otherwise, you may find yourself trying to pull back in your shoulders, producing tension and stresses in your back and running the risk of developing back pain. Of course, by the end of pregnancy, if you have to pick anything off the floor you'll be grateful for the exercise and the habits which have led to good lifting technique.

Do remember during this stage to maintain not only adequate rest but also to continue the particular relaxation techniques you've practised. By doing this your body will be well prepared for labour and you should be able to stay fairly relaxed throughout. Your labour will be easier, and your recovery smoother the more you're able to relax.

## Conclusion
Although obtaining the right amount of exercise in pregnancy requires a little thought, we hope that the guidelines given in this chapter are sufficient to enable you to obtain the right amount and type of exercise for you and your pregnancy. Remember too that

exercise isn't just for the pregnant woman. After your pregnancy it's still a good idea to take regular exercise. Moreover, it's not just you that can benefit. Your partner, too, may benefit from joining in with at least some of the exercises. And as your children grow up, they too may learn from your example, and adopt a healthy pattern of eating and exercise.

# 9

# Getting The Balance Right

**Making adjustments to your programme if you are putting on too much weight**

You should be monitoring your food, exercise and relaxation habits, using your diary. What happens if you discover you are keeping to all your mini-goals but your weight isn't quite right? The most likely problem is that you will be adding just a little too much fat. How do you stop this?

If you are putting on too much weight there are three different courses open to you. You can either cut down on what you eat, or increase your exercise, or a bit of both. Which course of action you choose will depend to a large extent on your stage of pregnancy. If it's the first trimester you may feel very tired and therefore it will probably be easier for you to cut down a little on food rather than increase your exercise. If it's the third trimester you'll probably find you feel just too big to increase your exercise, and so the only thing you'll be able to do is adjust your eating. Please remember, though, that you are not supposed to be cutting back too much on what you eat. You are supposed to be eating sound, well-balanced meals which will provide all the essential nutrients for you and the baby. You are not supposed to be going hungry to the extent that you are losing body fat. Equally, you should not be overeating. If you are putting on too much weight you are obviously taking in too much food and you should cut back to a more acceptable level, enough to maintain the medically recommended weight gain.

But perhaps you decide that you don't want to cut back on food at all. You won't put on excess fat if you use up all the calories you take in. If you are in the middle trimester doing more exercise might be your particular choice. However, it is worth noting that increasing activity is unsafe in certain circumstances. If your blood pressure is high, or at any time when you are even mildly ill (for example, if you have a cold), do not consider doing extra exercise. If there are any medical reasons whatsoever why increased activity (or, indeed, any activity at all) is to be avoided, then do not decide to exercise more and chance it. You will have to cope by eating just a little less instead.

For those of you who do decide to increase your daily activity in order to control your weight, you'll probably want to know just how much extra you should do. The best way of finding out is to do a little extra and then see the effect that this has on your weight over a few weeks. If you continue to put on too much, then you'll know you still haven't got the balance right. If your rate of weight gain becomes acceptable, then you'll know you are doing the right amount of exercise for the amount of food you are taking in.

It is possible, though, that the curious amongst you will still wish to know a little more about the calories that exercise requires. For many years dieticians have claimed that doing exercise is just too slow a way in which to control weight by burning up excess calories or stored fat. You'd have to walk a very long way indeed to burn off, say, 7 lb (3.2 kg) of surplus fat, whereas a standard slimming diet might get rid of this in about 3 weeks. This is very true. The only problem with this is that many people do not like going hungry, and never manage to keep to a slimming diet for longer than a few days. Also, with many of the very fast diets there is a real danger that you will lose lean muscle tissue as well as fat. If, after the diet, you put on weight again (and if you do not exercise), then the chances are that you will put on fat and you will not replace the tissue you have lost. The whole effect, after a few cycles of severe dieting and then overeating, is to make your body look very podgy. Without your clothes on, your body will look distinctly unfit and unfirm.

So, if at all possible, having exercise as at least a part of your weight control programme is generally a good idea. As a rule, the more strenuous an exercise is, the more calories it will burn up. A slow walking pace will use up about 2 calories a minute. A comfortable pace will use double this, and a very brisk pace might need 6 calories or more a minute. Brisk walking uses about the same calories as slow jogging, so if you feel too self-conscious to jog when you are obviously pregnant, walking is just as good. Swimming uses between 5 and 10 calories a minute, and so does cycling. The harder you work at the exercise, the nearer to the 10-calorie mark you come. You can see that any exercise that involves you moving your whole body about, which really gets the circulation going, will use lots of energy. You might think you're likely to burn off lots of calories by doing a morning's housework, but this isn't necessarily the case. Doing ironing, or washing up the dishes, or cleaning out cupboards, might use less than 2 calories a minute. This is because you're basically using only arm movements. You are not moving your whole body around at any pace at all. Housework may make you tired but it's unfortunately not very good exercise!

So doing a little extra of the *right* kind of exercise might be a very suitable way for some people to control their weight, some of the time (provided there are no medical reasons why they should not do this). Be careful here, though, not to overdo things. What if your calorie counting spotcheck reveals that the reason you are putting on too much weight is that you are eating around 1,000 calories too much each day? Instead of taking in around 2,400 calories, you are having 3,400! Don't even contemplate trying to fit in enough exercise to burn off an extra 1,000 calories a day. You aren't in training for the Olympics. You will simply have to cut your food intake to around the right level. You may decide to have about 2,600 calories a day, and do a little extra exercise to make up for the extra amount of fuel you are still taking in. This is fine if you feel you can manage it.

**What to do if you are not putting on enough weight**
A very obvious solution to this problem is to eat slightly more. We are assuming that there are no medical complications and the baby is developing well, but that you are using up your own body fat rather than relying on food to give you enough fuel each day. Generally speaking, unless you are grossly overweight, you should not try to have a very restrictive diet if you are pregnant. And if you are very overweight you need specialized advice from your doctor. Never just decide that you will be very severe with

yourself and try to follow a slimming diet in pregnancy. Look back at Chapter 4 and remind yourself of the right kinds of food to eat. Plan some exciting menus to tempt the appetite a bit. If you're feeling sick for much of the time, plan lots of small meals and snacks rather than fewer, larger meals.

Should you exercise less in order to save fuel and put on more weight? This is not a particularly good idea. Exercise has a lot more value than just using up calories! Done in the right way, exercise makes a very important contribution to health and general well-being. But what you could do is to keep your exercise how it is at present, *and* include more relaxation periods in the day. Don't be forever jumping up from your seat and rushing around doing little jobs. Take time off to lie back and do nothing.

## The importance of small changes in everyday life

Something that it is useful to remember is that in order to gain 1 lb (around ½ kg) of fat you need to overeat by about 3,500 calories. Similarly, to lose 1 lb (½ kg) of fat, you need to do without 3,500 calories.

You are very unlikely to be overeating by as much as 3,500 calories in any one day. This would mean you'd be eating 3,500 calories plus your normal amount (say, 2,400 calories), totalling 5,900 calories in one day. Most people could not manage this. And it would be virtually impossible to undereat by 3,500 calories in one day. If you normally need 2,400 calories, but you ate nothing at all, the most you could do without is 2,400 calories. This is equivalent to losing just over ½ lb (about ¼ kg) of fat. The scales might register a bigger loss, but this will be loss of water, and also could be partly due to the fact that you aren't carrying any bulk in your intestines, because you didn't eat for a day! As soon as normal eating resumes you will regain all but that ½ lb (¼ kg) or so.

The moral of this story is that it is difficult to make any significant changes in your body fat stores in any one day, or indeed, in any one week, no matter how hard you try. Even if you starved and ate nothing for a whole week, you wouldn't lose much fat. If you normally need 2,400 calories a day, then after a week of not eating you would have done without 7 x 2,400 = 16,800 calories. This means you would have lost about 4-5 lb (around 2 kg) of fat. You may have quite a large water loss from body tissues, but this will be replaced as soon as you start eating normally. You may have lost a little muscle tissue as well as fat, which is a bad thing. You will feel weak and ill and could well have endangered your health. If you did anything like this when you were pregnant it would be very bad indeed for the baby. Drastic action of any kind is not needed in order to control weight. Everything should *not* be done in a day, or a week, or even a month. The idea is make very tiny changes in everyday life. Make the changes so small that you hardly know you are doing them. They should be so easy that you *can* do them every day for months or even years.

When you are pregnant you won't be losing body fat, but you shouldn't be putting it on either. The fact is, you'll need to eat 3,500 calories on top of your pregnancy calorie needs in order to gain 1 lb (½ kg) of fat. You might think it's unlikely that you'll overeat by 3,500 calories. If you are weighing every day you should easily spot if too much weight (extra body fat) is going on. You'll be able to make the slight adjustments necessary to get back to target, before things get of hand. Remember that women who finish their pregnancy grossly overweight must have been eating a tremendous amount to accomplish this. To put on 20 lb (about 9 kg) of *fat* during pregnancy (*as well as* 20 lb or 9 kg of pregnancy weight) means overeating by 20 x 3,500 = 70,000 calories altogether. How do women manage to do this? Well actually it can be all too easy if it is spread evenly over the 40 weeks of pregnancy. The little changes (or even the little mistakes), if you make them every day, mount up to enormous changes after 40 weeks. If a woman overate by just 250 calories on each day of the pregnancy, this would equal 70,000 calories in total, and she would gain 20 lb (9 kg) of surplus fat which would be with her after the birth. This just shows how careful you must be to keep a watchful eye on weight throughout the pregnancy, and make the tiny adjustments needed to get weight right as soon as you notice that things are going wrong. If this woman had cut her calories by 250 a day, she would have put on no surplus fat. This is such a small amount of calories she would probably not have noticed much difference at all in her daily eating. Much easier to do this than to finish the pregnancy horribly overweight.

# 10

# After The Pregnancy

**Returning to normal: how long does it take?**
You should lose weight fairly rapidly when the pregnancy ends.
On the day you give birth you will lose the weight of the baby,
plus the amniotic fluid ('waters'), plus the placenta ('afterbirth').
This should total around 11 lb (5 kg). You will also start to lose any
extra fluid in your tissues; blood volume will start to decrease.
You'll lose about 6 lb (2.7 kg) in the week after the birth (mostly
because of loss of extra fluids and decreasing blood volume), and
then another 1 or 2 lb (½-1 kg or so) will go in week 2. By the end
of the second week the womb will have returned to almost its
original size and you won't be able to feel it in the abdomen. If you
still have a little pouch on your front this isn't the womb. It might
be partly fat if you have gained too much weight. And it might also
be partly due to poor muscle control, indicating a need for toning
up those abdominal muscles. If you haven't put on extra fat during
the pregnancy, your abdomen should be flat by the sixth week
after the birth. The exact length of time will largely depend on the
action you take to get all the relevant muscle groups toned up.
  You may have chosen to breast feed, in which case your breasts
will become very much larger in the second or third day after the
birth. Breast feeding may be very painful at first but you should
find you adapt relatively quickly, so that quite soon it becomes
completely painless. A fair trial would be to breast feed for around
4 weeks; by then, but probably much sooner, you should feel
quite comfortable and settled in your breast-feeding routine, and
be able to continue with it for as long as you wish. However, your
breasts will remain a little larger, and therefore heavier, whilst you

are feeding the baby yourself. For your own comfort it is essential that you obtain a good bra to support the breasts during this period.

You can see that if you have gained just the minimum medically recommended amount of weight (20-22 lb; 9.1-10 kg) your figure will very quickly return to normal, but with slightly larger breasts if you are breast feeding. However, because you look much as you did before you were pregnant, this does not necessarily mean that your body has fully recovered from the pregnancy. It might take some months before your body has completely readjusted and if you are breast feeding it will probably be about 2 or 3 months after milk production has ceased before you are back to normal.

The body takes time to readapt to its non-pregnant state. Do not necessarily expect to feel just like the old you in the few weeks (or even months!) after the birth. Of course, how you feel will depend partly on the kind of birth you had. A very easy birth can be expected to be less of a drain than a complicated or traumatic delivery. Some women *do* recover very quickly, and resume a normal level of physical activity within a few days of giving birth. This is fine if you genuinely are not tired and feel capable of it. However, this might well not be the case. In most hospitals women are advised to get out of bed, walk around, do a few easy post-natal exercises (for example, to tone the abdominal muscles) fairly shortly after the birth. This is probably all that most women will be able to manage without becoming excessively tired. You may have had some very ambitious plans about the exercise you would do once you'd had the baby, but don't be surprised if you are just unable to do much for a while. This may be partly due to lack of sleep. Young babies need to be fed remarkably frequently. Every four hours through the day and night isn't at all unusual. It could easily be far more often than this to begin with. You may cope well for a week or two but after a while you may become absolutely exhausted.

If this happens (it doesn't happen to everyone though) you must try to readjust your plans to fit in with the baby's own pattern. If the baby is fed and is asleep, you go to bed as well. It doesn't matter if it's daytime, if you're tired you must try to sleep. If you already have another child (or children) at home you will have to try even harder to find time to relax or sleep. It might well be that the only solution is to ask someone else to take the older children for the odd afternoon so you just have the new baby to cope with. Keep housework to an absolute minimum and, if possible, get someone else to do it for you. Keep meal preparation as simple as possible. Cold food (such as salads or sandwiches) can be just as nutritious as hot meals. If you can afford it, use disposable nappies for the new baby. These will obviously be the very small size of nappy in the period just after the birth, and these work out remarkably cheaply. If the brand you have bought seem to leak, check first of all that you are putting them on correctly (are they fastened up tight enough around the legs?) If this seems all right but they still leak, then try a different brand. Even if you have already bought traditional towelling nappies, why not start to use them later, once your baby is sleeping through the night and you have more energy and more inclination for washing and drying nappies every day?

If you do feel tired in the weeks immediately after the birth, do not be surprised by it. It's quite normal. The good news is that it doesn't last. Usually, by the time the baby is 6 or 8 weeks old, there are fewer feeds during each day and you should be getting more sleep. Your pattern of daily living should become a little more organized.

## Nutritional requirements after the birth

Your requirements will vary, depending on whether or not you are breast feeding. If you decide not to breast feed, then your need for nutrients will be roughly the same as before your pregnancy started. You will not need to eat extra. However, you should still continue with the low sugar, low fat, low salt, high fibre way of eating. This is the healthiest way to eat for everyone (including your baby, when he or she graduates from special baby milk and baby food preparations to a more complete diet). Your meals and snacks should remain, basically, a mix of proteins (from animal and plant sources), vegetables and fruit. You will need less of certain nutrients (such as calcium) than when you were pregnant. But you should find you are now less hungry, you'll therefore eat slightly less, and automatically the level of nutrients you take in will fall a little to meet your non-pregnant needs. If you are eating well, as we have shown you in Chapter 4, there will be no fear of running short of essential nutrients whether you are pregnant or not.

What if you decide to breast feed? You will need about 500 calories a day extra to the number you required when not pregnant. This is an even greater number than the 200 or so extra calories a day you needed when you were pregnant. But please do not think that these extra calories can come from just any food. Your need for vitamins, minerals and protein is extremely high and you may not obtain adequate amounts if your diet is high in sugary, fatty foods. As in pregnancy, it is best to let natural appetite be your best guide in choosing from nutritious foods high in protein, vitamins and minerals. You will probably find that breast feeding makes you very thirsty, so drinking plenty of skimmed or semi-skimmed milk is one of the best ways of ensuring adequate nutrition.

After about 6 weeks or so, many women start to introduce the occasional bottle feed because they fear they are not producing enough milk. This is very unlikely indeed. You will not run out of your own milk, provided you let the baby suck as often, and for as long, as he or she requires. The more sucking that occurs, the more milk is produced. Occasionally, a baby may cry for a feed very frequently, perhaps every hour. Provided you let your baby feed this often your milk supply will increase to meet the demand. This might well be the prelude to the baby sleeping through the night. The baby may need about three or four feeds during the evening, 'stoking up' in readiness for a full night's sleep with no milk. This pattern should only last for a relatively short while. You will eventually find a more leisurely routine establishes itself, whereby the baby normally demands milk just five or so times during the day, and then sleeps through the night.

If you do introduce bottle feeds, the baby is sucking at the nipple for less time. The less sucking that occurs at the breast, the less milk you will produce. So, as soon as you start to introduce bottle feeds, your body will automatically readjust and produce slightly less milk. This, of course, is fine provided you want to discontinue with breast feeding. You will need to eat less food if you are producing less milk. Again, natural appetite should be your best guide. Do not eat if you are not hungry.

## Reducing your weight after the pregnancy

With luck, there should be no need to reduce weight after you've had your baby. If you've followed the advice we've given you, then you should have added no surplus body fat and you'll be right back to a good shape within a few weeks of the birth. However, if you've miscalculated slightly, you may have put on a little fat. Perhaps you had to cut out your exercise right down at some point, making it harder for you to control your weight. Or, maybe you misjudged how much food you needed for a few weeks, and by the time you took corrective action you'd put on some unnecessary weight. Anything up to about 7 lb (3.2 kg) of surplus fat isn't at all unusual.

In the past many women have gained a little fat with each pregnancy, and never lost it. Although 7 lb (3.2 kg) isn't a great deal to add on, it mounts up if you have more than one pregnancy to make a decidedly plump figure. It is wrong to assume that you will naturally weigh more just because you've had a baby. You must make every effort to lose your extra weight, even if you only weigh a little more than before you were pregnant. It's unhealthy to be overweight, and a little fat seems to lead inevitably to a lot more fat as the years go by, UNLESS you take immediate action.

If you weigh too much, the questions you'll want to ask are, how soon can I start a diet after the birth? And, can I diet if I am breast feeding, or should I wait until the baby is weaned? What we strongly suggest is that you start to lose your extra fat *immediately* you realize that you are carrying too much. If you have only a little fat to lose, you'll probably have to wait a few weeks after the birth before you realize that you're not quite as slim as you were. But, if for some reason you've put on far too much fat, this will probably be apparent very quickly after the birth. So, if you are too fat you must take immediate action to lose this. But what should that action be? What you absolutely must not do is to start a strict, very low calorie diet after pregnancy. You are in for a very busy and possibly tiring time, and you need to eat properly in such circumstances.

You must plan to lose your extra weight in a slow, systematic way. Aim to lose weight at a rate you feel comfortable with. We suggest no more than 2 lb (about 1 kg) a month. Firstly, let us consider how to lose weight if you are breast feeding. You will be needing about 500 calories a day more than you did before you were pregnant. If you normally used to need 2,200 calories a day, you now will need 2,700. So, to lose about ½ lb (¼ kg) a week, you'll need to take in slightly less than this, about 250 calories a day less in fact. Therefore, if you ate 2,450 calories a day you would lose around ½ lb (¼ kg) a week. Alternatively, you might have a full 2,700 calories, but exercise more (for example, briskly walk an extra 2 or 3 miles every day). Or, you could balance the food and exercise together; walk just one extra mile and have about 2,600 calories a day. You'll know when you have got all this adjusted right, when you see the scales register an appropriate drop in weight.

We're not seriously suggesting that you count every single calorie and do exact amounts of exercise in order to lose weight. But we've given you this example in detail just to show you how *little* you have to do in order to lose ½ lb (¼ kg) of fat a week. The tiny changes you make to your diet and your exercise routine really add up to enormous changes in your appearance and health. To try a diet regime of 1,000 or even 1,500 calories a day is far too restrictive for most women to stick to, especially whilst breast feeding. Even if you are very fat, reducing your calorie intake to. below 2,000 a day is nearly always unnecessary if you are producing milk for your baby. It could well make you hungry, depressed and run down to drastically reduce calories. So don't do it. However, you do need to boost your morale by knowing you are doing *something* towards controlling your weight. A ½ lb (¼ kg) loss a week may not seem much, but you'll lose about 13 lb (5.9 kg) if you continue losing weight like this for 6 months.

Breast feeding your baby can be a remarkably time-consuming thing. You might feel like eating a meal, but then the baby starts to cry and your own meal is delayed or even forgotten about. Some women find that, whilst actually feeding their baby, their own appetite disappears. For such reasons as these, it is very frequently the case that the mother simply doesn't take in quite enough food each day and therefore uses up her own fat reserves. For a great number of women, breast feeding leads to extremely easy weight reduction. It's slow, it's steady, and it's safe, provided that when you *do* eat, it's from a wide selection of good, nutritious foods. Don't try to lose weight faster than around 2 lb (1 kg or so) a month.

We have already shown you some methods of weight control, like using your diary, noting your daily weight, making out graphs and charts. Continue to do this if your weight isn't yet back to normal. You should now be quite good at interpreting your daily weight and you should therefore be able to see if your weight is going slowly downwards. If it is not, simply eat very slightly less each day. Perhaps you could do without that extra slice of buttered toast at breakfast, *or* go without a similar amount of food at any meal. Eating just a little less and exercising just a little more, should soon result in the drop in weight that you desire.

If you are not breast feeding your baby and you are overweight, or if you have finished breast feeding but are still a little overweight, then what should you do? In theory, there is no reason why you should not follow a standard slimming diet, provided that it is based on sound nutritional principles and it is not too severe or restrictive. If you feel you can follow such a diet successfully then give it a try. But if you break your diet and stop losing weight, OR if you are successful in losing weight but then you put the weight back on again, do not carry on using standard slimming diets. Please don't become a 'yo-yo' dieter, going on and off diets for years and years and never achieving lasting success.

Instead, use the methods we have already outlined in order to lose your weight. Concentrate mostly on good nutrition rather than cutting down too much on food. You need to retrain your eating habits permanently. Make sure your diet is low in fat, sugar and salt, and high in fibre. Try to lose weight at around the rate of 2 lb (1 kg) a month. This only means having about 250 calories less than you need each day. If you normally have around 2,200 calories a day, have about 1,950 instead. You could step up your activity slightly as well if you like. You don't want your metabolism to slow down so that you only need the 1,950 calories you are taking in! It might be a little difficult to organize free time for exercising once you have the baby, but going for brisk walks is always possible if you push the baby along in a pram or buggy; you'll both benefit from the fresh air and sunshine. Remember, to lose 2 lb (1 kg) of fat in a month isn't much, but this is 24 lb (around 11 kg) in a year, and 48 lb (around 22 kg) in 2 years. Such a loss should solve most people's weight problem. To take a year or two to slim is a relatively very short time compared to all the rest of the years you will live, without having to bother with diets, and with no weight problem. Most people are at least a little overweight for many years, if not for their whole lives, because they never find the simple and easy method of weight control.

## Other weight problems after pregnancy

It's just possible that you carefully controlled your weight during pregnancy, but after the birth you relax a little too much and add a little weight. Perhaps you might tend to continue eating the same amount you needed when you were pregnant and therefore put on fat. This is a real danger for women who bottle feed their baby. Some women find it especially tempting to overeat once they start their babies on solid foods; it's very tempting to finish off baby's leftovers. It's important to remember the things you learned about weight control through your pregnancy. The principles you picked up then should become second nature to you. Even without keeping a diary, if you just don't eat unless you're hungry, you should stay slim. Your baby will fast become a toddler. This will, in itself, introduce a fair amount of activity into your day. It should help to keep you slim. As far as your child's food goes, be careful to give him or her healthy, well-balanced meals. If you are not giving your child lots of sugary foods, it would be unfair for you to eat them, wouldn't it? Your child should prove to be one of the best ways of controlling your own weight that there is!

Perhaps, though, your problem isn't that you are too fat, but that you have become a little thin. If you are just a little underweight, do not worry too much. Provided you are eating nutritious food, the weight will probably go back on when you are a little less fatigued with looking after the new arrival. It's essential that you do not skip meals. Try to get extra help from friends and neighbours if you feel it's all getting too much for you. Incorporate more relaxation periods into the day. If you're feeding the baby, sit down, put your feet up, and try not to think about anything taxing or worrying. If you're breast feeding you'll probably become thirsty so have a *cold* milk drink whilst the baby is taking his or her meal. (Note, though, NEVER have a hot drink whilst you are feeding the baby; if you spill it the baby may be severely scalded.) You might like to keep a pile of magazines by the chair in which you feed the baby. You may not want to focus on the baby all of the time, and he or she can get on with the job whilst you read something lighthearted and entertaining!

## Permanent weight control

Using the methods of self-control we've outlined in this book, anybody should be able to become exactly the weight which is healthiest for them, both during and after pregnancy. They can do this by adopting a better way of eating and by incorporating more activity into their daily life.

To begin with, you will need to use a diary, a weighing machine, and all the other tools and methods we described in Chapter 6, in order to control your weight as you wish. However, with the passage of time, these external aids should become unnecessary. You will learn to appreciate the internal cues which tell you that you have a genuine appetite for something. You will also learn to recognize the internal sensations which tell you when you've had enough to eat. You will get used to leaving food when your appetite is satisfied. After a while you'll find that your body feels stale unless you do exercise regularly. When all these things come naturally to you, you'll know you've acquired permanent weight control.

# Further Reading

E. J. Bassey and P. H. Fentem *Exercise: The Facts* Oxford University Press, 1981.

G. Bourne *Pregnancy* Pan Books Ltd, 1979.

G. Cannon and H. Einzig *Dieting Makes You Fat* Century Publishing, 1983.

P. Fisher and A. Bender *The Value of Food* Oxford University Press, 1979.

A. Maryon-Davis and J. Thomas *Diet 2000* Pan Books Ltd., 1984.

M. Polunin (Ed.) *The Health and Fitness Handbook* Sphere Books Ltd., 1983.

If you follow a vegan diet, then useful information can be obtained from the Vegan Society, 33/35 George Street, Oxford, OX1 2AY.

# Index